YAEL DREZNIK

Battles in White

Yael Dreznik
Battles in White

The story of the medical, nursing, and rescue teams on the 7 October attack

I wish this story would never have been told.

Table of Contents

Table of Contents

Prologue

When the first words of this book were written, we were still counting our dead. The most murderous terrorist attack that occurred on the soil of the State of Israel began on the morning of October 7, 2023, as the sun rose on the second holiday of Sukkot, the Simchat Torah holiday. Thousands of terrorists infiltrate into southern Israel under the cover of a coordinated missile attack, massacring about 1,200 people— residents of the south, soldiers, civilians. They beheaded, raped, amputated limbs, tortured, burned to death, and took more than 250 people—including babies and the elderly, women and children—into Hamas captivity.

The element of surprise and horror left the State of Israel in terrible shock. The fact that exactly 50 years earlier, the State of Israel was caught by surprise in the Yom Kippur War only added to the incomprehensible dimension of the failure, of concepts that collapsed into themselves as the separation barrier itself collapsed between Gaza and Israel.

Nearly 70 years ago, in 1956, Ro'i Rothberg was murdered in Nahal Oz, a kibbutz near Gaza. He was 21 at his death and left behind his wife and infant son. Terrorists from Gaza entered the kibbutz, murdered him, and mutilated his body. On his grave, the then Chief of

Staff, Moshe Dayan, delivered one of the most famous eulogies in the history of the State of Israel. Reading the words today is chilling.

"Early yesterday morning Roi was murdered. The quiet of the spring morning dazzled him and he did not see those waiting in ambush for him, at the edge of the furrow. Let us not cast the blame on the murderers today. Why should we declare their burning hatred for us? For eight years they have been sitting in the refugee camps in Gaza, and before their eyes we have been transforming the lands and the villages, where they and their fathers dwelt, into our estate.

It is not among the Arabs in Gaza, but in our own midst that we must seek Roi's blood. How did we shut our eyes and refuse to look squarely at our fate, and see, in all its brutality, the destiny of our generation? Have we forgotten that this group of young people dwelling at Nahal Oz is bearing the heavy gates of Gaza on its shoulders? Beyond the furrow of the border, a sea of hatred and desire for revenge is swelling, awaiting the day when serenity will dull our path, for the day when we will heed the ambassadors of malevolent hypocrisy who call upon us to lay down our arms.

Roi's blood is crying out to us and only to us from his torn body. Although we have sworn a thousandfold that our blood shall not flow in vain, yesterday again we were tempted, we listened, we believed.

We will make our reckoning with ourselves today; we are a generation that settles the land and without the steel helmet and the cannon's maw, we will not be able to plant a tree and build a home. Let us not be deterred from seeing the loathing that is inflaming and filling the lives of the hundreds of thousands of Arabs who live around us. Let us not avert our eyes lest our arms weaken. This is the fate of our generation. This is our life's choice - to be prepared and armed, strong and determined, lest the sword be stricken from our fist and our lives cut down.

The young Roi who left Tel Aviv to build his home at the gates of Gaza to be a wall for us was blinded by the light in his heart and he did not see the flash of the sword. The yearning for peace deafened his ears and he did not hear the voice of murder waiting in ambush. The gates of Gaza weighed too heavily on his shoulders and overcame him." (From the eulogy).

On the morning of October 7, 2023, we did not see the terrorists lying in wait for us along the boundary line. In a meticulously planned and demonic act, babies, children, teenagers, women, men, grandfathers, and grandmothers were murdered. They were the citizens and soldiers who went to build their homes and their outposts at the gates of Gaza, to be a wall for us. The light in our hearts blinded our eyes, and we did not see the lightning strike of the enemy. The longing for peace deafened our ears, and we did not hear the sound of the lurking murder. The gates of Gaza were too heavy for our shoulders, and they overcome us.

This is the story of the medical, nursing, and rescue teams on the most terrible day that befell us, on the State of Israel. It is the story of medical heroes, encompassing endless dedication and sacrifice under fire, in one of the most unbearable, mass casualty events in human history — and medical history.

This book is dedicated to them.

8

Chapter 1: Trip to Vienna

"Do you have a balcony?" Rotem asked me the day before we met. "Because it requires a cigarette; my story."

Rotem Zelman has been a nurse at the Sheba Medical Center, the largest medical center in Israel, for over ten years. She spent years working in the surgical department, learning how to treat wounds, and provide care for patients with various types of injuries.

She completed an intensive care course and became an integral part of the trauma team. In other words, being a trauma nurse means being a trauma coordinator who is able to coordinate various trauma events, including road accidents, gunshot wounds, terrorist attacks, and mass casualties. This role requires composure and high coordination skills. One must know all the relevant procedures, mediate between them all, and understand the combination of injuries and different trauma conditions in neurosurgery, orthopedics, or general surgery.

We met when we were at the beginning of our professional paths, in room seven of the surgical department, at the start of my internship as a doctor. Rotem wanted to learn how to insert an IV and asked me to be with her in the room, along with a hospitalized patient, a nice grandmother we were learning on. A squirt of blood and an eventually successful IV insertion marked the beginning of a long and shared journey of ours.

Over the years, as she advanced and grew from a nurse in the surgical department to a skilled nurse in intensive care unit and trauma, she also tried to mediate several personal traumas in her private life. An indistinguishable mix between her two parents who died, within an unimaginable time span of only a month, just when she had prematurely born twin daughters. She intertwined personal tragedies with the blood, sweat, and tears of the surgical department.

Still, she says, on her fourth cigarette on my balcony, sometimes even when you think you're an expert in trauma coordination—

there are moments when you're not.

They're a tight-knit family, Rotem's family. After all the personal tragedies—the parents who passed away one after the other, and the other blows that befell the family—it was clear they would rise, meet every week, and become even more bonded than before. This was both because their numbers had dwindled and out of a need to preserve the tradition even more.

Medical and nursing professionals work on this at home too, not just in advising friends and family members on any medical case, no matter how trivial. They are also the ones who sometimes need to bind everyone together, like the biological glue used to adhere wounds. It means being the ones who know how to bandage the family's wounds, of the sister, the brother, the relative. It's also about setting an example for Rotem's niece, Shira, who wants to be a nurse. Something about this profession makes people look at you and tell you how much they want to do what you do. And that's what Shira wants to be, exactly like Rotem.

Shira is a soldier in the army, about a year into her service, around the beginning of October 2023. She's an observer at the Nahal Oz base - a soldier tasked with preventing infiltration attempts and attacks on Israel by entities- like terrorist- located near the country's borders, through the use of computerized tracking systems.

She's the eldest daughter at home, has long hair and ocean-blue eyes, and she knows she's the eyes of the state, that she and her friends see what's happening at the border and warn against the enemy, and truthfully, she feels a great sense of mission. Not every girl dreams of being an observer before she joins the army. Many of these would-be soldiers don't even know what it involves at all. But during the course and training, the recognition that it's a role with significant importance solidifies. A role that can save lives. Shira's team at the base calls her "Shira, beloved by the terrorists," because she always managed to prevent infiltrations and warned in advance about dangerous events.

A while ago, there was a story about someone from the Gaza Strip who put an unidentified object on the the fence that constitutes the border between Gaza and Israel, and Shira got everyone on alert, and in the end, it turned out to be a watermelon, and how she felt embarrassed about that watermelon story, and only relaxed after the commander praised her for her alertness and caution.

When you're a soldier in the army, nothing is really certain. You try to maximize your time, those moments when you're suddenly at home, with the family. Sometimes everything works out, the vacations align well for everyone, and then you go abroad with the family for a specific week, say, the first week of October. And sometimes you decide to travel the week after.

And Shira is exactly planning a trip with her family to Vienna on the first Saturday of the Sukkot holiday.

When we have children serving in the army, especially in combat units, there are moments when we wonder why they volunteered for such dangerous combat roles instead of choosing safer positions, like observation, similar to Shira's role.

And there are moments when we think otherwise.

Sukkot has just begun.

Sukkot is an excellent holiday for traveling abroad, coming after Rosh Hashanah and Yom Kippur. There's at least a two-week gap during which the children are not attending schools and kindergartens, and we haven't really started the year with all its daily burdens and chores. There's still time for family vacations, even though we've just finished July–August. This period is especially perfect for soldiers to travel with their families, who are exactly on break, right before training or after completing a course. Everything aligns so that Shira finds the perfect time, after a year of basic training, courses, and military service, to travel with her family — with her mother, who is Rotem's sister, her father, and her younger brother — to Vienna. Just before the trip, she applies pink nail polish, a luxury for soldiers finally on a short break from the army, hastily taking care of themselves in the hours, days, and moments they are not bound to uniforms, weapons, and standard appearances, a polish that even prompts Shira's father to ask if it's allowed.

Simchat Torah- the last holiday of the beginning of the year- is just around the corner, the days pass lazily, with not even a hint of rain yet. Many families choose to leave home for tents outdoors, camping across the country, or taking a break abroad — prices are always higher, and flights are accordingly expensive, making all camping sites full to the point that it's hard to find a place in such a small country.

Rotem finishes another day of work at Sheba, in intensive care, happy that her sister and the kids are back from Vienna. Her young daughters are very attached to Shira, and almost every time she comes back from the army, they see her. However, this time, because of the trip to Vienna, they didn't get to see each other.

This is a transitional period, just like the holidays themselves. At Sheba, they plan to move into a new, secured intensive care unit. Everything is ready for the preparation and integration; the move to the new and equipped ICU is supposed to happen within a month. No one knows exactly when it will take place, but the transition requires a lot of preparation. In addition to working in intensive care, Rotem is undergoing additional training as a trauma nurse, planning to complete another course and to get training at another hospital. Everything is still relatively fresh, and there's so much more to learn.

"I remember how I was with you once in a MCI (mass casualty incident)," Rotem suddenly throws us several good years back. "I remember how you and Gravitz treated a bleeding wounded person, everything was one big chaos, you barely managed to put on gloves," she recalls.

A mass casualty incident (MCI) is the most defining event for any hospital, anywhere in the world. Any other event — a big concert, school opening, a ceremony with many participants — is such that preparations are made weeks, months, and even years in advance. But a MCI in a hospital is very hard, if not impossible, to truly prepare for. Occasionally, medical teams undergo refresher courses- declaring an MCI day, wearing special uniforms, treating simulated casualties, drawing conclusions, and preparing for the real moment. However, when the real moment arrives, it tears up all the plans.

When we think about MCIs, we primarily consider two different types of events in their nature and the types of injuries involved throughout human history. One type is a natural disaster, such as an earthquake, tsunami, or hurricane. These events are almost impossible to defend against, if at all, and include various physical injuries, including drowning as a result of submersion, different crush injuries, burns, etc. Among natural disasters, earthquakes accompanied by tsunamis

— like those that occurred in the Indian Ocean in 2004, claiming the lives of more than 270,000 people — are considered the deadliest in earth's history, and the ability to anticipate and prepare for them on a medical level is almost nil compared to the force of nature.

The second type of mass casualty incident is one that humans are responsible for, such as terror attacks, battles, and wars. Human history is rife with blood-soaked MCIs caused by humans, and the last few decades have seen several such events etched into global consciousness. The Twin Towers disaster, or more famously known as 9/11, is perhaps the most well-known example of an MCI.

Sheba medical center is a tertiary trauma center and the largest hospital in the country. Trauma medicine, in general, is divided into primary medicine, i.e., the initial assessment and treatment given to an injured person, for example, by the ambulance care team. Secondary medicine is essentially treatment by a specialist, i.e., the injured person being transferred for treatment by a specialist in orthopedics, for example. Tertiary medicine offers not just specific specialization but highly specific sub-specialization. For instance, an injured person needing not just an orthopedist but one specialized in spinal surgery. Hence, a tertiary trauma center like this can provide cutting-edge medical treatment to every trauma patient, equipped with the facilities and capabilities to offer such advanced care.

Rotem is accustomed to the beeps of her pager announcing incoming patients to the trauma ward, and sometimes several injured patients together who need to be prioritized. Yet, she knows that despite the countless events she has already participated in, involving severe traumas, an MCI can occur at any moment and shake the professional ground she stands on. However, she doesn't think about this daily. Trauma team members don't dwell on such significant events in their regular routine; it's something hard to comprehend and grasp.

The information and experience accumulated among trauma experts regarding MCIs have led to the development of extensive literature, attempting to organize all knowledge in a way that enables efficient event management. There's even a special chapter on MCIs in surgical textbooks, which begins with "An MCI is a risk that always exists, and therefore, every medical team member and medical system must be prepared." In this context, two critical points are essential for understanding an MCI. The first is that such an event requires preparation for a large number of severely injured patients who need rapid and immediate assessment. The second is the importance of triage, the initial sorting. This role requires a skilled team member to stand at the entrance to the triage area or in the zone where the injured are received and decide within seconds who is lightly injured, who is moderate, who is severe or critical. Who needs surgery now and who can wait for a structured assessment in triage.

Although there's a multitude of injured people with severe injuries in most mass casualty incidents, it's usually the less severely injured or those suffering from anxiety who arrive first. Therefore, conducting triage professionally is crucial, as it distinguishes between well-managed and poorly managed events.

The term "triage" originates from French. Napoleon's surgeon, Baron Dr. Dominique Jean Larrey, recognized the importance of identifying the most severely injured as a priority. The concept of triage began on the battlefield in the 18th century, where the initial sorting of the wounded took place within the battlefield itself, in Field triage. The definition of an MCI is very broad, ranging from an event with just a few severely injured individuals to an extreme event reported as a disaster, i.e., an event where the hospital's ability to treat injuries is always lacking, and the staff is exposed to grievous injuries and total destruction. Between all these definitions, different treatment principles have been learned through experience — sometimes unsuccessfully. For example, one that emphasized the importance of safety among caregivers in hostile territories, or errors in treatment that should never happen, or the significance of having an incident manager and the need for available blood products at all times.

But no one thinks about an MCI during the holiday. It's the end of the week, Thursday, October 5, 2023, and Rotem is mainly happy about having a quiet weekend at home with her husband and her twins. Her sister always travels on Saturdays to visit Shira, in Nahal Oz, with tasty food, pots, and home-cooked meals, but this time, after the family returned from Vienna, they decide to stay at home and spend a few more days of longing.

Chapter 2: Uninhabited land

Sukkot is about to end, and with it, the return to routine. We celebrate it in memory of the Hebrews who left Egypt after a long period of slavery. According to the Hebrew bible, they wandered in the desert for 40 years and resided in temporary shelters called sukkot—not quite a house nor a tent, but a structure that simulates the feeling of home, with walls, linens, and a roof of branches above.

At the end of Sukkot, the Jewish people celebrate Simchat Torah—a holiday that is dedicated for completing the reading of the Torah over the year and starting anew. The last portion read on this festive day, just before starting again from Genesis, tells of Moses' death, how the leader of the Hebrews ascended Mount Nebo, gazed upon the Land of Israel, and peacefully passed away, leaving behind his blessings.

Just as Moses led the Hebrews through an uninhabited land, Dr. Ella Shaier, who moved to Israel from Russia at a young age, chose to settle in Mitzpe Ramon, a place located in the desert, among the dust. "A child who moves from another country doesn't truly grow roots," she explained to me, "perhaps only in such a place, where the desert mountains envelop you in a tranquility that makes you truly feel at home." From a young age, she fell in love with the desert and stayed there from the first moment. Ella is a senior physician, an emergency medicine- E.R specialist for several years. From a young age, she knew she wanted to be a doctor, but the paths, like the place she chose to live in, were not paved. Initially, she was a paramedic, then studied medicine in Hungary, completed her residency in internal medicine at Soroka, and then considered studying emergency medicine.

As odd as it might sound, the field of emergency medicine is relatively new in Israel. It's an established field for years in other countries, but in Israel, it only gained recognition as an independent specialty, that of emergency physicians, in the last decades. These are the doctors who need to handle hundreds of stressful situations daily, those who must quickly identify which patient is deteriorating and why, seeing those who come to the emergency room at their most critical moment, the moment when one of the most important things in medicine must be done: make a decision. And make a good one.

"Somehow, I feel most at home in this profession," she says. "I manage to stay calm under pressure. It puts me in a mode of action where I feel most comfortable."

When she decided to study emergency medicine, it was precisely when the profession was just beginning to stand on its own feet. And it seemed to her again like an uncultivated land that needed to be walked anew and for which principles and rules had to be established, like-what is an emergency medicine doctor, anyway? What are their areas of responsibility? What are the boundaries within which they operate? But today, it seems that everything is clearer. The rules have been established, there are new initiatives all the time, and there is unique training. To be a doctor in emergency medicine and understand this dynamic called triage, one needs to be familiar with the world of internal medicine, the surgical world, spend part of the time in intensive care, and know pediatrics.

The training program accordingly is diverse and includes various rotations, that is, medical experiences and medical training in several different sites in hospitals, not just in the emergency department (ED) itself. To earn the title of an emergency medicine specialist, one must complete training lasting several months in an internal medicine department, in an intensive care unit, understand the dynamics of the operating room and trauma room, etc. The skills required of an emergency medicine physician include not just rapid diagnosis in triage but also initial treatment in triage before being admitted to a hospital ward, to surgery, or to intensive care, such as medication balancing, bedside imaging, suturing, initial orthopedic response, and even performing resuscitation and treating advanced shock.

It's a kind of work that hardly ever has a moment of rest. Every doctor at the beginning of their career who has done shifts in the ED remembers that moment when suddenly time passes so quickly, the feeling that hours just slipped away, due to the fact that it's such an intensive place.

Unlike all other medical specializations, the world of the ED cannot be neatly defined with a beginning, middle, and end. It's not like a surgeon, for example, who sees a patient needing surgery, operates on them, sends them home, and sees them afterward in the clinic. Or like an internal medicine doctor in an internal medicine department, who treats an inpatient, medically balances them, cures them, and sends them home. Being a doctor in the ED—or, in general, being a team member in the ED—means that for that team member, the beginning and middle are clear, but the end is often shrouded in mystery. What happened to that patient who arrived in the middle of the night with pneumonia and was admitted to the hospital? And what eventually happened to the woman who was injured in an accident and we sent for surgery? It's a world where primacy stars—the initial diagnosis, the initial treatment, the initial medication—with big question marks about the end. Those that caused me, as an intern, to walk around with patient sticker's names during my rotation in the ED, just trying to close the circle, to find out what became of my patients.

Being an emergency medicine professional requires certain qualities, such as the desire to rush to a new patient, to reach a preliminary diagnosis as quickly as possible, and to know how to properly triage, to understand where the patient belongs, under which medical definition they should be categorized. For example, a 70-year-old grandfather who arrives at the ED confused, is he suffering from an acute infectious process, or a cerebral event, or alternatively a problem with his salt and electrolyte balance? The focus of emergency physicians is the correct placement of the patient in a differential diagnosis definition, combined with the ability to draw conclusions quickly and coherently—qualities that Ella felt she had, fitting for this special occupation.

Ella lives in Mitzpe Ramon with her husband and children, and she works at Soroka. She travels to work every day, an hour there and an hour back. Often, she travels in the dark, for the night shift she regularly mans on certain days, and then returns to the escapism offered by the desert. "Here you won't hear sirens," she says, "if there was ever a siren here, it was probably by mistake."

I imagine that bridging between the silence of the desert and the countless events in which Ella was involved in trauma management at Soroka is probably achieved only by an hour's drive on roads enveloped by desert dust. She regularly works the Saturday night shift, arriving at ten in the evening and leaving on Sunday morning, and works two more nights a week, plus a full day of work. Generally, the way of working in the ED is very unique and different from what exists in regular hospital wards. Given that it's such an intensive place, there's also significant burnout, and it's important to know how to preserve the workforce and allow for moments of respite.

Ella, in her role as a senior doctor at the largest hospital in the southern region of the country, sees everything that the emergency department of a large hospital has to offer: a bustling ED with elderly patients from nursing homes, young people after road accidents, individuals arriving with severe abdominal pain or excruciating headaches or terrible back pain, stabbings and injuries, falls and cuts, bloody urine and swollen abdomens. And the ED always knows how to surprise; there's always a special case that deviates from the usual routine. A case that we remember and tag in our medical and human memory.

Soroka is not just a hospital with one of the busiest emergency rooms in the country; it's a medical center that provides primary care to the population in the southern region of Israel. Among its many units, advanced institutes, and departments is the Pediatric Intensive Care Unit (PICU), one of the most complex and emotionally taxing places for medical staff. Dr. Eitan Ne'eman is a senior doctor in the PICU, and on that weekend, he is on call at the hospital, planning to make a visit on Saturday morning as well.

"Eitan and I met at the age of 23. He had just finished his military service in the navy and was debating whether to start studying medicine and improve his matriculation exams, or to stay in the navy, with the religious world also pulling him in. Despite all his deliberations, it was clear to me that the world of medicine suited him more," tells me Yael, his widow. She tells me about the young Eitan, who was then a naval officer. He decided to become a doctor after an inspiring encounter with a pediatrician who did his military service on the ship where he served. Yael and Eitan met through a mutual friend, and within a year they got married, settled in the south of the country, close to Soroka Hospital, and had seven children.

Eitan was clear about his desire to be a pediatric intensive care doctor. For pediatricians, specializing in pediatric intensive care is considered one of the most challenging specializations. It combines several difficulties simultaneously — emotional difficulty facing the families of small patients who are a hair's breadth from death, physical difficulty due to the scarcity of experts in the field, which necessitates many on-call shifts, and cognitive complexity from the need to deeply understand various physiological mechanisms and pathologies at a very fundamental level, and to make quick decisions.

"Already during his medical studies, in his fourth year, Eitan decided to specialize in pediatrics. His love for the demanding field of pediatric intensive care, which requires a specific subspecialization after completing pediatrics, began when he was a young intern, meeting Dr. Tzachi Lazar, who would later become the head of the PICU. He did a rotation in the PICU very early on, during 11 night shifts a month," Yael continues, "After completing his pediatrics residency, he began his fellowship in pediatric intensive care at Yale University Hospital in Connecticut, three not easy years that advanced him medically but deepened his longing for Israel."

When they returned to the country, Eitan began to thrive. He promoted projects at the hospital, such as resuscitation exercises.

"The day before October 7, we happened to hear the song 'On the Launch Line', and we talked about how it was our song, about how Eitan reaches new distances in the race, and I am still on the line- watching him and waiting to join my own race, but mainly seeing how my partner reaches professional heights," tells me Yael.

"He managed to combine his expertise at Soroka with volunteering in the army in two combat units — the 669 Search and Rescue unit and the 551 Commando unit — while simultaneously volunteering to give lectures and continuing education for Magen David Adom crews, and in a civilian rescue unit in Arad. He spoke Arabic with an amazing level of proficiency, with an accent. He was much more than a promising professional doctor. He was enlightened. He had the ability to give families the feeling that he was there for them all the time," she adds, "He wanted to promote multidisciplinary care for patients who were determined to be brain dead. He felt that the families of these patients needed to receive a strong and supportive envelope that would continue to accompany them, which is much beyond what only a medical team can provide."

24

Pediatric intensive care personnel, like emergency medicine personnel, are exposed to the most difficult sights there are and need to pick themselves up each time anew, mainly for the sake of the patients, but also for their own. The ability to give, to heal, depends on our ability to first deal with ourselves, with the way we tag the difficult events we treat. This tagging of special and difficult sights in our memory, us healthcare professionals, sometimes leaves scars. And the constant engagement with human tragedies, under pressure and anxiety, can scratch us, sometimes for a limited time and sometimes forever. Over the years, the scars fade, and the emotional deposits make room for the capacity to encompass. The freshness always characterizes the beginning, like the anxiety I felt when I saw, as a student, the morgue before the dissections in the anatomy class, metal gurneys on which lay bodies wrapped in blue blankets, the strong smell of formalin, rapid heartbeat from the very sight of death so tangibly. Or like the experience you go through when you see a resuscitation for the first time, or when you announce bad news — all these things remain in memory as a base on which equally shaking experiences are laid, but those whose cumulative effect over the years is such that it is possible to live alongside it.

Some studies conducted on medical teams in cases of difficult events found that the group with the greatest resilience — those who are able to emotionally deal with an event in the best way — is the group of doctors. After them, are the nurses, who also know how to cope with difficult sights and heart-wrenching stories. The weaker groups are those that are in action, more on the periphery rather than at the center, such as the janitors, for instance.

The fear is that these workers will develop acute stress disorder or anxiety disorders. But in the end, no one is really immune. I understood this fact, that no one is truly immune, myself, during my first resuscitation as an intern in the internal medicine department, when I heard from the outside the shattered cries of the family, when the whole corridor was filled with people I did not know, exactly at the moment when we were supposed to come out and announce the death of a patient. I felt it also in other cases, like in a case of a young woman who came to the emergency room complaining of coughing, and without prior preparation, I discovered that her chest X-ray was filled with metastases. To this day I won't forget the moment when I came out of the X-ray room and her daughters smiled at me, sure that it was just pneumonia. But even when I thought I was really immune — because those events touched me but I continued to walk in an orderly trajectory, one that allows me to process them and continue and advance — there were still those cases that scratched, perhaps irreversibly. Like the beeper that announced a severe road accident, two years ago, after which I was called to the trauma room to treat a boy who was riding a scooter and was seriously injured. A short round of resuscitation, dilated pupils, and a cold body of a 12-year-old boy, and I declared death. It was not the first time I declared death in my life as a doctor, unfortunately, there were too many moments of declaring death before, but it was the first time I felt how something wounded me and did not heal afterward, in the moments when I held the mother hugged together with me, and took her to identify her son. And the resilience washed away from me, maybe it faded and strengthened intermittently, but it never really returned.

In recent years, there has been a growing recognition of the critical importance of the mental well-being of medical teams worldwide.

Programs and protocols to maintain the resilience of the teams started to emerge worldwide, including in Israel, with Soroka, the largest hospital in the Negev, being the first to launch a resilience program for its employees. The goal is to identify the distress of hospital workers in advance. To identify the doctor who cannot sleep at night after a difficult experience with a patient. To talk to the nurse who has been complaining for two weeks about a lack of appetite and penetrating thoughts following exposure to difficult sights in the emergency room. To arrange a meeting with the sanitation team responsible for the morgue, for example, in the case of a mass casualty event.

Iris Raz is a senior nurse at Soroka, serving in several roles, including midwife, psychotherapist, and head nurse in Soroka's resilience unit. She began her career as a midwife, later engaged in psychotherapy, and moved to coordinate the response in the hospital's resilience unit: the unit for supporting medical teams. She is 64, married with four children, has lived in the Negev all her life, and is very familiar with Soroka, through all the operations, security events, and wars. "The hospital is very practiced in mass casualty events," she says. "we have people who are skilled in managing events with many casualties, everyone knows their role, where the command center is, what everyone needs to do." She has been operating, along with Dr. Yael Levaot, the head of the hospital's resilience unit, the emotional support for hospital teams for three years, and over the years, the skill and ability to identify potential emotional issues in advance have developed.

"In the beginning, after we deal with difficult events, there are reactions that seem normal," she says. Professionally, this phenomenon is called Acute stress reaction, characterized by difficulty sleeping, lack of appetite, and concentration issues. When this condition lasts more than a few days, it becomes a medical issue, and the precise term is Acute stress disorder. "To me, these are warning lights," Iris explains. "It's about people who are constantly under pressure, report difficulty concentrating, can't sleep, wake up in the middle of the night — and then we come into the picture."

The idea is to raise awareness of the phenomenon, to talk, to provide initial help. When we manage to properly treat it — to give that person the feeling that it's reversible, that we can help — we can try to prevent the progression to Post-Traumatic Stress Disorder (PTSD). PTSD is so named when the symptoms become chronic, i.e., last more than a month. It is already a disorder that can severely impact quality of life, expressed among other things by night terrors, mental distress, avoidance of any event that may remind of the trauma itself. And it's worth remembering that the disorder can occur not only in those who have experienced trauma but also in those who treat someone who has experienced trauma, and here the resilience unit of Soroka comes into the picture.

But it's Friday evening, 6.10.2023, and there is no hint in the air of trauma, catastrophe, absolute evil. It's a holiday evening, and Israel is savoring these moments to the fullest, before the holidays end and a long period of routine begins. And on that Friday, we — I, my husband, and our youngest daughter, Nitzan — are traveling to Kibbutz Dafna, right across the border with Lebanon in the north of Israel. We leave at home our older daughter, Tamar, who returned from the army and is meeting her boyfriend, Gal. Tamar is in the midst of an officers' course as a combat soldier and is supposed to receive her placement later on, and I am meanwhile trying to suppress the fact that my daughter is in a life-threatening role. I am mainly happy that ahead of me is a quiet weekend. There are no duties or night shifts at the hospital, just quality time with my family by my side. We just hope we manage to sleep properly in the tent, along with hundreds of families around us.

At the same time, as the sun sets on Friday, Iris and her husband are in the north, near the Sea of Galilee. She plans to swim a bit in the morning, and then to travel back south to Be'er Sheva. They are hanging with her husband's friends from the army — he still volunteers in a central role in the reserved army in the Southern Command, responsible among other things for evacuating casualties, despite having passed the age of reserves long ago. They sit down for dinner with all the friends and celebrate the holiday evening. A few hours later, he will wake up early in the morning and tell her, even before it all begins, that he has a bad feeling.

And in Mitzpe Ramon, at that time, Ella's husband is putting the children to sleep, as every evening since the beginning of their relationship. She has a quiet evening and a quiet morning afterwards, contemplating what to do the next morning, making herself an evening coffee, reading the newspaper, with the sky outside clear and strewn with stars. This sight always reminds her of the great advantage of the desert surrounding her.

And when the skies are so bright, and all of Israel sits in sukkot and tents, between the streams and on the seashore, and when the laughter

29

of children fills the camping sites and the kibbutz lawns, and celebrations of Simchat Torah with its processions are planned for the next day, we believe we have already seen everything and we are rich in experience from being the State of Israel, accustomed to suffering, wars, rounds of fighting, and rockets.

But we haven't seen a thing.

Chapter 3: Fake news

Magen David Adom (MDA) is the national emergency medical service of the State of Israel, and as of 2023, it operates approximately 1,400 ambulances, of which 300 are mobile intensive care units. The range of MDA's roles is extensive, including not only pre-hospital emergency medical services but also blood services (including donation, testing, and distribution of components), first aid training, and humanitarian activities. Additionally, MDA serves as Israel's Red Cross society.

MDA, like all emergency organizations worldwide, determines the required level of readiness for each day, which is usually updated according to the readiness level that is declared by various security services, military forces, or police forces, as needed. As such, staffing levels, both at the service center and in ambulances in the field, are not full since, on an average day, only about 300 rescue vehicles are needed rather than a full staffing. This means that at the station itself, there is a team that rotates every eight hours, like hospital nursing shifts, and includes ambulance drivers, paramedics, and sometimes even doctors. When an increase in the level of readiness is required— for example, If there is an escalating security event or an alert about a large event with many casualties, the organization's readiness level is raised to match the threat level.

In extreme cases, the readiness level is raised to full staffing, meaning all positions, motorcycles, ambulances, mobile intensive care units, and various rescue vehicles are fully staffed, 24/7. Such a situation is common in wars and is not frequent.

Saturday, October 7, is a holiday. At the end of the day, celebrations are planned in synagogues, around the Torah scroll. The morning hours are summery, the evening before is a holiday eve, and many families gather for full family meals. MDA does not receive an alert about an especially unusual security event. That evening, a concert by the artist Bruno Mars is supposed to take place in Tel Aviv, with tens of thousands of participants, but beyond that, the area is quiet. Apparently, there is no reason to raise the readiness level higher than usual, but a decision is made at the management level of the organization to raise the readiness level to level B. The implication is full staffing of about half of the rescue vehicles, twice as much as on a regular day. It is due to the large number of people expected in the public spaces during the holiday, the heavy movement of travelers, extensive cultural activity, and concerns about a possible attack.

Saturday morning, 06:29 a.m. For millions of people in the State of Israel, in hindsight, this exact hour will be remembered as an eternal turning point, a border line stretched between the world that was and the world that now is. Like an alarm siren symbolizing what was about to befall us, a siren shatters the morning in many areas across the country. In other places, people wake up to reports from friends or family members, while rescue personnel are awoken by the annoying buzz of their beepers.

On Saturday morning, October 7th, at 06:29, a surprise attack by Hamas and other Palestinian terrorist organizations commenced from the Gaza Strip onto Israeli territory. Thousands of rockets were fired at various regions across the country, from the south to the north, including the central area. Many Israeli citizens woke up to the sound of alarms and entered safe rooms or shelters, while others were updated on the extraordinary attack through the "Red Color" alert applications.

Dr. Rafi Strugo, a specialist in internal medicine and emergency medicine, who has served as MDA's chief physician and Deputy Director General of Medicine, also woke up to the sound of the alarms, understanding that this was an extraordinary event. He felt the event was exceptional for two main reasons: firstly, it was not preceded by any warning. Unlike previous security events, which were usually preceded by warnings of an escalation, here the surprise was complete, foreboding ill omens. The second reason that hinted at an unusual event was the significantly exceptional intensity of the rocket fire compared to previous known events. The MDA dispatch centers are already receiving calls about rocket impacts in various places and about casualties and even fatalities caused by the massive rocket fire.

The CEO of MDA and the organization's management were already at MDA's national center, beginning to manage the response to the many calls flowing in. As minutes passed, it became apparent that under the cover of the massive rocket attack, Hamas members and terrorists from the Nochba (Elite) unit breached the fence at the Gaza border in several places under the cover of the massive rocket attack, rushing toward Israeli territory, specifically to the southern communities and IDF posts, armed with massive amounts of ammunition.

At MDA's dispatch centers, isolated calls about gunfire heard in several places began to be received. "In those moments, one of our senior managers, who lives in a kibbutz near the Gaza Strip border in the south, directly contacts the chief executive officer of MDA"- Dr. Strugo recounts, "he updates that there are terrorists at the entrance to the kibbutz, and that the team has been alerted." The report itself sounded so unrealistic — terrorists at the entrance to a kibbutz? Terrorists on the fences? "No one believed it was something that could happen," he notes, "certainly not on such a scale."

As minutes passed, it became increasingly clear that the rocket fire was a relatively minor distraction in a monstrous and deadly event. Under the cover of massive rocket fire, thousands of terrorists infiltrated Israeli territory, particularly the southern communities adjacent to the Gaza Strip, gradually taking over the southern settlements. MDA's dispatch centers began receiving dozens of calls from residents of various communities in the surrounding area reporting injuries from gunfire and terrorists roaming the settlements and on the roads. MDA's first teams send out to these events — some of them were injured themselves by terrorist gunfire — and they too reported encounters with terrorist cells in different places in the area. In various WhatsApp and TikTok groups, videos of terrorists driving and shooting in all directions, storming doors, and carrying RPG missiles began to circulate. It was so imaginative at first, that many of us didn't really believe that this was what was happening on the ground.

Dr. Yoram Klein is the director of the Trauma and Critical Care Surgery unit at Sheba Medical Center. Sheba is also a Level 1 trauma center, similar to a few other major hospitals in the country, such as Soroka, the largest hospital in the Negev, capable of providing all the necessary medical response for trauma victims. This definition is important for understanding a mass casualty event and the world of trauma in general, even in cases of a single injury. To receive the standard or definition of a Level 1 trauma center, a hospital must have surgical residents available around the clock, an available team of anesthetists, emergency medicine specialists, neurosurgeons, orthopedists, plastic surgeons, and oral and maxillofacial specialists, among others, but not exclusively. This definition should be given to a hospital that regularly treats a certain minimum number of trauma patients. A hospital that does not meet these requirements cannot be considered a Level 1 Trauma Center. This does not mean that such a hospital cannot treat trauma patients, but there are cases in which the hospital will not be able to provide the appropriate response, for example, in situations involving head injuries that require neurosurgical intervention not available in all hospitals. In such cases, when a patient arrives at a hospital considered Level 2 and, for example, needs neurosurgical intervention, a transfer to a Level 1 hospital will be coordinated.

Dr. Klein has been involved in trauma for many years, a unique field in general surgery that requires extensive knowledge in physiology and the various body systems and the ability to make quick decisions. "I actually have been dealing with trauma since the moment I operated on the first soldier who came to me as a casualty in the 90s," he recalls.

Doctors choosing to specialize in general surgery usually select their subspecialization and further specialization only during their residency. Some decide to focus on transplant surgeries, others on oncological surgeries, and so on. Dr. Klein chose general surgery because he wanted to deal with trauma long before his specialization. Throughout his years working as a traumatologist at Sheba, he has developed and expanded the trauma unit, so today it also deals with other critical conditions requiring surgical management.

His counterpart is Batya Segal, a trauma coordinator nurse at Sheba, and one of the most experienced nurses in the hospital. Batya came to Sheba at the age of 18, still as a military nurse, and advanced from a nursing degree to various roles in the surgical departments and the intensive care unit, until she finally became the trauma coordinator. Among their responsibilities as trauma providers are coordinating, providing, and transferring trauma patients.

When people think about trauma specialists, they often envision a scenario where a patient is brought to the hospital, and a trauma specialist jumps on them immediately, performs invasive procedures, such as inserting chest drains, central venous catheterizations, intubations, etc., and rushes to the operating room. In reality, the role of a traumatologist is fundamentally different. He manages the event, a well-defined role in all trauma textbooks. When the patient arrives, the trauma manager is responsible for a team that includes other doctors and nurses, primarily focused on understanding the situation, i.e., reviewing the monitors' readings, receiving updates from the team on the patient's physical condition and injuries, and making decisions.

In such a situation, the traumatologist typically stands aside and does not participate in the various procedures his team is performing during the assessment in the trauma room. His role is to process all the information within a few minutes and decide on the treatment approach. When the patient is unstable, the decision may be dramatic - it can range from an extreme situation, such as stopping resuscitation and declaring death, to deciding whether to perform advanced surgical procedures in the trauma room, such as emergency thoracotomies or urgent preperitoneal packing if the patient is in deep shock or losing vital signs.

When the patient is stable, the decision includes the type of imaging to be performed and the location best suited for the patient after the preliminary assessment, such as an operating room, intensive care, or hospitalization in the surgical ward.

Putting traumatologists in this position - supposed to stand apart - allows them to process data very quickly and from an overall perspective, but that's not always possible. In some situations, the traumatologist is the most qualified to perform certain life-saving procedures because he or she is the senior surgeon.

For instance, a few years ago, when I was on duty in the emergency room, and Dr. Klein was my trauma on-call, the beeper went off: "A 60-year-old man, riding a scooter, arrives with severe head, abdomen, and chest injury." Within minutes, one of the most severe casualties I had ever treated was brought into the trauma room, suffering from a severe head injury, dropping blood pressure in front of our eyes.

There are moments as a surgeon that I vividly remember. Whenever I close my eyes, I can see the scene in my memory again - a 60-year-old man unconscious, sedated, and intubated, with a massive hematoma in the pelvic area. In the trauma room, I recall Dr. Klein realizing that this patient had arrived with a crushed pelvis and was bleeding into his pelvis and about to collapse, and that he, meaning Dr. Klein, was the only one in the room who knew how to perform an urgent pre-peritoneal packing- a lifesaving procedure.

I also remember the exact words he told me when we opened a surgical kit for a pelvic opening- "Dreznik, cut here, like in a C-section, don't injure the bladder"," the noise in the room that didn't bother either of us, the nurses bringing special pads that were filled with blood.

Also, I recall how quickly and methodically Dr. Klein placed the pads into the pelvis until the bleeding stopped, so we could relax.
As someone who performs countless shifts a year, Dr. Klein is accustomed on a daily basis to making such life-and-death decisions, of which action to perform and why, of the correct order of actions.

In the morning of October 7th, 2023, He is awakened by the sound of an alarm. Within minutes, he understands he has to go to the hospital, to Sheba. However, he also receives other messages, horrifying ones- such messages that deviate from the usual confrontations.

"I'm receiving videos that are circulating on Telegram and the network, and from friends, about terrorists driving tenders through Sderot," he says. "I am 100% convinced that it is psychological warfare - there is no way these are real reports."

Dr. Klein's partner holds a senior position in the Israel Police. While Dr. Klein does not believe the videos circulating online, she is already receiving messages about a real concern that terrorists have infiltrated Israeli territory. At 07:11, she texts him that the army has activated a special code, reserved for such events. The implication is clear: there has certainly been a terrorist infiltration, and it's a combined attack of rocket fire from the air and a ground operation on a scale that is still unknown at this stage. "Still, I can't believe it's real," he says, "she sends me a video of a terrorist's driving in Sderot next to a police car. I was sure it was fake news."

Meanwhile, at MDA's headquarters, preparations are underway to make decisions whose outcomes are translated into several directives on the ground. The first order is to dispatch more than 20 bulletproof ambulances southwards, capable of entering areas where there is concern about terrorist infiltration. The second order is for full staffing of all ambulances, "an order that was last issued only during the previous war," Dr. Strugo adds. The third directive is to staff all the telephone dispatch positions to handle all incoming calls.

Such a call comes to an MDA dispatcher. One of many calls.

A young boy, nine-year-old Michael, and his younger sister, five-year-old Amelia, are in one of the southern kibbutzim, witnessing the murder of their parents before their eyes, and they also manage to see their three-year-old sister running to the neighbors. Both run to the safe room inside the house and decide to call the police. Half an hour later, when the police do not arrive, the children call MDA, where a dispatcher connects the call to Linoy, an MDA paramedic.

"I answer the call," Linoy recounts, "and suddenly I hear a child's voice telling me he's calling for his parents and they're not answering, that he thinks they're dead. He understands that he's now responsible for his younger sister and is in an impossible situation. I tell him to yell loudly for his parents, if they respond, I tried to understand through the phone if they are salvageable, and I quickly realized that the focus needs to be on how to save these brave children, who are in immediate life-threatening danger."

Linoy, the paramedic talking to the children on the phone, asks little Michael to move to the safe room's door and lock it. He tells the paramedic that he is also looking after his younger sister and that he is struggling to close the door. Linoy instructs them to get inside a closet, she asks if there is a closet in the safe room, and tells little Michael that help is on the way.

"Don't open until good people come," Linoy says, and instructs him to call the dispatch every time he is scared. And he did call. Time after time. Hour after hour. Two small, frightened children, hiding in a closet, for 14 hours. Without food. Without water. Without parents.

Thousands of calls arrived at the MDA dispatch that day. All of them a desperate plea for help, a request for rescue and medical care.

Medical forces try to reach. The first MDA ambulances were dispatched at seven in the morning in Ofakim, a southern city about 30 kilometers from Sderot. The station received a call to treat five shooting victims in the junction area, and on their way there, suddenly four motorcycles and trucks loaded with terrorists came within a few meters of one of the ambulances.

Initially, no one thought these were terrorists, who from a distance and in motion looked like soldiers. Even when they shot at the ambulance driver, it took a few minutes to understand the significance of shooting at an ambulance. Another ambulance driver, who was also rushing to the junction, was murdered by terrorists shooting at him.

As the minutes passed in the morning hours, it became apparent that the rescue forces faced an impossible task. The entire area was threatened by terrorists who had taken over the territory and were moving from house to house, murdering entire families, and taking control of traffic routes.

As ambulances tried to reach the area, they encountered police and military roadblocks that prevented them from reaching the area, forcing them to divert victims from other locations, some of whom arrived independently. The scene began to look like one of the scenes of a massive mass casualty event.

Chapter 4: They knew their job

The Gaza Strip is a coastal strip of land near the sea, covering an area of about 360 square kilometers, approximately seven times the area of Tel Aviv, and as of 2023, it has over 2 million residents. Gaza has been the source of terrorist attacks almost continuously since Israel's establishment. The kibbutzim and towns close to the border with the strip have suffered for many years from various terrorist events, from harassments and infiltration of terrorists.

Even within the Gaza Strip, before the disengagement from it, Jewish settlements - the Gush Katif bloc - suffered from intensified terrorist events. In 2005, the disengagement plan was decided upon, and as part of it, IDF forces withdrew from all areas of the Gaza strip, and all Israeli citizens were evacuated from it. The border between it and the State of Israel was closed, and the territory was transferred to the exclusive control of the Palestinian Authority. In 2007, Hamas forces took over the Gaza strip. The Hamas regime led to an increase in rocket fire and many military operations in response. Naturally, the communities close to the border absorbed most of the different terrorist actions: infiltrations of terrorists, incendiary kites, and the burning of thousands of dunams of fields and forest trees, as well as rocket and mortar bomb launches.

Noam Esh Zuntz is a medical student living in Sa'ad, a pastoral kibbutz near the Gaza border. Sa'ad is a beautiful place- with green spaces and garden apartments, and beautiful landscape that has accompanied her since childhood. "At 06: 30 in the morning, we wake up to an endless barrage of launches. I have never experienced such in the 30 years I've lived in the kibbutz," she tells me. She ran to the safe room with her two young children, Jonathan and Tamar, and with her husband, who serves as an officer in the Air Force.

"We hoped the children would not wake up from the alarms, but both of them were immediately awake and ready. We closed the safe room door and explained to three-year-old Jonathan that there are booms outside, so we stay in the safe room that protects us." Meanwhile, outside, the barrage doesn't stop. The kibbutz receives a message that there are injured in the clinic, that everyone should stay in the safe room, lock doors, close and darken the windows. Along the way, Noam's mother calls and updates that the house of Noam's 90-year-old grandmother was hit directly, and then she says that terrorists have infiltrated from Gaza, breached the fence. "When I see that my mother also sent a message, it becomes even more frightening, and I don't really understand what's happening."

Noam has not yet completed her full medical training but feels she must help in any way possible. She texts the kibbutz nurse and asks if help is needed in the clinic, and the nurse responds that they have moved from the clinic to the nursing home opposite to accommodate all the injured. "Don't leave the house," the nurse tells her, "it's dangerous outside. We're managing for now." Within half an hour, that nurse would learn that her son's phone, who lives in kibbutz Be'eri, has fallen into terrorist hands. It would take her a week and a half to find out that her son was murdered, ten days of utter lack of information and pure terror. "I'm frustrated that I can't help," Noam tells me, "I know there are several gunshot wounded, but I trust our nurse in the kibbutz that she's managing the event and can help."

Staying in a safe room feels suffocating. A safe room, or a fortified space within a residential apartment, is designed to offer protection against missile attacks. I sometimes think to myself when I enter our home's safe room, normally the bedroom of our eldest daughter, that it is the only country in the world where people are required to have a gas-proof window, ventilation pipes, and reinforced concrete walls when they buy a house.

Noam and her husband minimize their constant use of the phone; but she has to text her sister who just gave birth a week ago and is already in great pain and stress. She's very worried about her, and meanwhile, they try to keep the kids occupied. Her husband builds a tower with magnets with their son, and she keeps their younger daughter busy with a ring stacker so she won't dismantle the other games, and "we even promised them we'd go outside to prepare for the Simchat Torah processions," she adds. While hearing gunshots as she walks to the bathroom but quickly returns to the safe room.

"My children are fed up, they're hungry and want to go out. They are kibbutz children, accustomed to open spaces and grass. And the hours drag on. We bring schnitzels and rice to the safe room, making an improvised lunch. I have no appetite for anything," adds Noam.

"Then I hear horrifying news about a party near Kibbutz Re'im, with people hiding in shelters into which grenades were thrown. And that the Nahal Oz base was captured. I hear that my cousin, who was just on vacation, killed a terrorist who entered the house of friends in his kibbutz, and that terrorists have taken over Kibbutz Kfar Aza, located just two minutes away. Terrorists are controlling Kfar Aza?"

Kfar Aza is the kibbutz across the street. They were there for countless joint meetings of children and families. Last monday Noam was there with her children in the orchard, and they enjoyed it so much they planned to return, and now? They understand they are under siege. Be'eri, Nahal Oz, Kissufim, Kfar Aza, and they are in the middle, next in line. In hindsight, precise maps of the terrorists were discovered, with clear sketches of where to enter, whom to kill, and how.

She spreads a blanket on the floor after managing to put the children to sleep for a nap. They have to leave the door of the safe room slightly open for air and light, her husband sits at the entrance to the safe room, guarding everyone, and Noam starts to cry.

Continuing south on Highway 232, one reaches several more settlements and communities that also belong to the the south Regional Council, which encompasses all the settlements close to Gaza strip. In this area, the Western Negev, there's a Magen David Adom first aid station located at the furthest point in the area. In remote stations, specifically this one, employees work in 24/7 shifts, and on that Saturday morning at six-thirty a.m., Menachem Blumenthal, a paramedic, is there with his ambulance driver, about to finish a 24-hour shift since Friday morning.

Menachem, 43, is married with five children and lives also in Kibbutz Sa'ad. After his military service, he earned a bachelor's degree in emergency medicine and has worked as a paramedic for over twenty years, also teaching emergency medicine. In the early hours of Saturday morning, he was looking forward to heading home to see his wife and kids - Simchat Torah was approaching, and he had had a relatively routine shift. "As a matter of fact, we even checked in on a party going on in Re'im during the night, ensuring everything was fine and nothing special was going on," he recounts. At large outdoor parties with thousands of attendees, there's always the potential for various medical incidents - dehydration, injuries, etc. - but there's an ambulance on-site for emergencies, so Menachem tries to catch a few more minutes of sleep before his shift ends.

Like Noam, Menachem and his driver wake up to the barrage of rockets. "We quickly receive a call about a severely injured person in one of the greenhouses in the area, due to a rocket falling," he says, "At that stage, we didn't know about the infiltration of terrorists, so I told my driver to take the main road, Highway 232, as quickly as possible, to pick up the injured and head to the hospital."
The driver, for some reason, suggests taking more side roads instead of the main highway. Alongside the main road, there are smaller roads, sometimes only well known to local residents. They might extend the route slightly, but they're less exposed. "His decision saved our lives," Menachem says. What they didn't know at that stage was that the main road was swarming with terrorists who had breached the fence.

"We pick up the injured worker, a Thai laborer, from the greenhouse hit by a rocket. He's in a lot of pain, with burns and wounds all over his body, and in addition, there's a language barrier, but somehow we manage and prepare to drive back to the hospital. Then our dispatcher calls us and says that the whole area is under terrorist infiltration, and that it's currently impossible to leave, but rather to treat the injured here, on-site."

How do you treat a severely injured person in the field, and how do you treat a severely injured person in an area threatened by terrorists? "We entered one of the settlements, to the study hall area, which seemed relatively protected. There was a fortified space in the area. We laid out our equipment, and we stayed there, alone with the injured. The feeling of helplessness was immense," Menachem tells me. It's impossible to comprehend what's happening, there's no way to know what to do, and medical care is unavailable to him. He repeats this several times. The feelings intensify each time an injured person arrives at the improvised corner for treatment in the settlement, from the very understanding that the way to treat them is limited. In the absence of an advanced set of treatment kits, or with a very small set that includes only an infusion, fluids, and a limited number of bandages, and without the ability to evacuate, there's a feeling of helplessness that is hard to explain how despairing it is.

So many other occupations today allow for a minimum of aids for work purposes. We live in a world where a bank account, a laptop, and an internet connection are enough to run a virtual office, make huge transactions, and provide diverse services. But when it comes to medicine, we return to the physical world, to medical equipment, and our dependence on it. This aspect was defining on that day of October

7th, echoing unanimously in every conversation with every team member who was in the field. With every paramedic who, other than holding the injured's hand and assuring that rescue is on its way, had nothing else to do.

Meanwhile, Menachem hears more reports: there is heavy fighting in the nearby area, and there are more injured who can't be evacuated to the hospital. They understand that they will serve as a holding station until it is possible to organize the transfer of injured to another place, and in the meantime, more and more injured arrive. And the injuries are severe. "They knew their job, the terrorists," Menachem recounts. The injuries are in areas not protected by the bulletproof vest such as severe gunshot wounds in the pelvic area, lower and upper limbs.

Menachem understands that if a helicopter doesn't arrive, the injured he is treating in the improvised holding area, in the study hall area of the settlement, might die. They were already treated with fluid infusions, plasma, painkillers. The local nurses join in too, washing the wounds. Human suffering is terrible. For instance, one of the injured arrives with amputations of both upper limbs. He tried to reach the fortified room when terrorists placed an explosive device on the entrance door, and it exploded on him. Another injured died despite all attempts to save him. A woman at the end of her pregnancy arrives in the area suffering from advanced labor contractions, and there's a discussion on how and whether to deliver her in the field.

"When I teach about emergency medicine, we always know there's a scenario where we need to treat the injured in the field—an extreme scenario where it's not possible to evacuate the injured. It includes opening first-aid warehouses found in every MDA station," he summarizes, "But no one ever dreamed in their worst nightmares about such a situation, we just improvised with what we could. Our ambulance went to bring injured and along the way to pick up medical equipment, and we tried to do our best. In the end, after a military helicopter arrived, rescue helicopters also came, which helped to evacuate the injured and the pregnant woman." And in a corner on the side, the bodies were gathered, and one of the community members was tasked with guarding them.

And when Menachem tells me about that community member staying over the bodies in the improvised hospital, as he and his team treat dozens of injured—it's beyond all imagination, beyond all nightmares. Or as Noam wrote to me, "All my memories are stained with blood. Will we ever have a home again?"

Chapter 5: United rescue

Avi Markus, a 46-year-old married father of five, is a professional paramedic with over 20 years of experience in providing advanced medical aid, including in medical helicopters, to patients with various degrees of injury. He is a volunteer at "United Hatzalah"- a first aid organization, which in recent years has been operating alongside Magen David Adom and counts thousands of volunteers, dozens of ambulances, intensive care vehicles, and medical evacuation helicopters.

Emergency medical services in Israel, as in any other place in the world, need to consider several critical parameters when deciding to evacuate an injured person to the relevant hospital. Every doctor working in an emergency department is familiar with the pager message from an ambulance updating on an incoming injured person, but a First aid organization needs to rely on prior considerations. For example, is the hospital equipped to receive an injured person with a specific injury. Another consideration is whether, as a result of transferring a large number of injured individuals to a particular hospital at a given time, the transfer should be diverted to another hospital.

In essence, the treatment of an injured person includes several variables, and there is critical importance to every stage of the process, from accurately connecting with the injured in the field to bringing them in an organized and coordinated manner to a treating institution that can admit them. This means knowing where to drop off the injured—whether it's the trauma rooms, the ER, or a special helicopter landing pad—who is waiting for them, and what information needs to be conveyed about them. In cases of multiple casualties, such as a severe road accident with many injured, communication becomes even more complex.

First aid organizations have an emergency protocol for exceptional events, with the fear of many injured, expressed in a system that broadcasts emergency reports to the team members. The likelihood of such a special broadcast occurring on a holiday morning without any prior warning is almost unimaginable. So imaginary that when Avi wakes up from the vibration of the communication device, he thinks there's a bug in the system.

When Avi wakes up, he sees a series of reports flooding the broadcast, about one shooting event after another and injured in different scenes in the southern part of the country. " I recognize that we're dealing with a mass casualty incident occurring at multiple locations." he shares. "It's clear to everyone that we need to start moving rescue vehicles south, the problem is that there are dangerous areas threatened by terrorists, so we're also taking extra precautions."

Avi isn't just a paramedic in United Hatzalah, a civilian rescue organization; he's also a reserve paramedic in a commando unit in the military, and he's well aware that it's only a matter of time before he gets called up for emergency duty. In the meantime, he's getting ready to head towards a gathering area in the south where rescue forces start to flow.

Like Avi, Hani also volunteers in United Hatzalah. Hani Vaknin, almost 40, is married and a mother of four. The eldest daughter is already 20 and has just gotten married. Hani works for a living as a supermarket manager and has been volunteering as an emergency medical technician (EMT) in United Hatzalah for more than five years.

A family tragedy inspired her to volunteer and has become one of her most fulfilling activities. This volunteering – going out of the house at least once a week, wearing the rescue uniform – is what allows her to look at life differently. "It's not just about putting life into the right proportions, it's also about showing your kids, your surroundings, that you're doing something good for others," she notes. " my kids see it, they are raised by the example of their mom."

On the morning of the attack, Hani wakes up at six-thirty to the sound of an alarm in her town. She's on duty that weekend, and with the first alarm, she still believes, like everyone else, that it's an isolated event, one without any medical implications, like many incidents of rocket falls in recent rounds between the State of Israel and the Gaza Strip that often ended with only property damage. When the second alarm sounds within a few minutes, it's clear to her that something else is happening here. Like Avi, she understands that this is an exceptional event, and she's getting ready to go out.

Both receive the information from their constantly flashing pagers, and it's clear to them that something significant is happening. But apart from reports of a large number of injured across various scenes in cities and kibbutzim in the south, the full picture is still missing. Hani takes her personal gun along with her rescue uniform and heads towards the ambulance. She meets her husband, just returning from the synagogue, informs him she is on her way to the south, to areas already reported to have dozens of injured. She is not afraid of the event itself. "I am going to do what I need to do. I hear there are injured children outside, and my children are safe at home, so I leave immediately and go on my way."

A bit further north, Noemie wakes up to the same alarm. Noemie Dray, only 27 years old, immigrated to Israel from France at a young age, lives with her parents, and is studying at a nursing school. Noemie began volunteering at emergency medical organizations at age 15 and later became an EMT in United Hatzalah, also coordinating the resilience program in her city. This special program, like the one at Soroka Hospital, aims to provide psychological support to victims of anxiety or shock, in situations requiring mental and psychological intervention.

Noemie recalls waking up to a flood of alarms on Saturday morning. "It was clear to us that this was something exceptional. The pager beeped, putting us on high alert and signaling the possibility of an ambulance being dispatched south." She is connected to her device at those moments, starting to receive pagers about the alert. "At this stage, all of us in the family, who are in the protected space, understand that this is something else," she says. The United Hatzalah ambulance stops by her house around 8:30 in the morning, and she gets on it along with the team that will accompany her, including the ambulance driver, a paramedic, and another EMT. Meanwhile, she says, while driving in the ambulance towards the south, reports start coming in about injuries to rescuers, like an ambulance driver shot in the head and an ambulance hijacked. At the same time, she hears about other surreal reports, like terrorists roaming in vehicles, armed, threatening the civilian population. "I think that at those moments, we hardly understood the situation, like the report we received from one of our coordinators, about another United Hatzalah team member who was shot in the head."

The radio is constantly busy, unending gunfire in the background, and the road to the south has never been more terrifying. "There was a lot of chaos; we felt like we were entering a war zone," she adds, "There were clouds of smoke all around, and suddenly, right before our eyes, we saw bodies scattered at the entrance to Sderot, a terrorist's pickup truck, gunfire in the air." At this stage, Sderot—the city closest to the border between Israel and the Gaza Strip—is under an infiltration attack by dozens of terrorists attempting to take over, among other things, the local police station. Many videos circulating at that time on various media channels show terrorists who have penetrated into the city of Sderot, whether it's footage of shooting and RPGs fired at cars near a neighborhood supermarket or incidents in the city's central neighborhoods. During the ground infiltration, the relentless barrage of rockets on the city is heard non-stop. "When we arrive in Sderot, we hurry to the police station there. We were updated that there's a gathering point, there were medical, military, and police personnel, and only two ambulances at that hour," she recounts. Meanwhile, wounded individuals from various places, some in critical condition and intubated in the field, are brought in military vehicles to the gathering point.

Into this reality—of injured people arriving from almost everywhere, of terrorists freely roaming Israeli territory, a reality that seems as if taken from a nightmare and at those moments not fully comprehended by most citizens of Israel—are exposed Avi, Hani, and Noemie, as well as hundreds and thousands of volunteers in the various rescue organizations, in those first minutes and hours.

The element of surprise always exists for anyone providing first aid. You never know whom you'll meet, under what circumstances, and in what condition. I never knew to guess—when I drew the curtain behind the bed in the ER, or when I received the call from the ambulance—who I would treat, where they were from, what they were doing moments before they were injured. Who is the person I meet in moments of sheer terror, even fear for their lives?. We also don't know the circumstances of the accident or event happening in a split second, including the kinematics or the type of ammunition involved.

Often, at the scene itself, bystanders try to tell us about the car that crashed with great force into the car beside it, about a motorcycle rider thrown into the air. These descriptions help us to form an understanding of the event's nature, including the severity of the injury. It's clear to us that when a child is thrown from a car several meters away, the injury is not similar to an injury from a collision between vehicles moving at low speed. And yet, even if we are familiar with various and strange mechanisms of injury, nothing prepares the rescue teams in the first hours of Saturday, for the reports they hear and the sights they see.

For example, reports of dozens of injured soldiers requiring immediate triage, which Avi begins to conduct in the gathering area, when suddenly a car stops next to him with two soldiers who appear to be sitting in the back seat. "But when I see them, I'm updated that these two young soldiers are dead," Avi recalls one of the most difficult and arresting moments of that day. "And I step aside for a moment and break down. I suddenly feel like I'm choking, remembering how I used to extract dead soldiers from a tank when I was a soldier in the army, and it all comes back to me, but I have to pull myself together and go back to doing triage."

Or, for instance, a report on a large nature party in Re'im, with a multitude of injured people of varying injury degrees. And to that area, Hani's ambulance arrives.

"Nova" is a music festival held at that time in celebration of the Sukkot holiday, in an open area near Kibbutz Re'im, about five kilometers from the Gaza Strip. Over 4,000 revelers were present at that time, and as the rocket fire began, the party-goers followed the familiar drill. The festival organizers abruptly stopped the party, and the attendees began to disperse, some by car, and some received messages about gunfire in the area that started shortly afterward and sought shelter in the surrounding bomb shelters. A video from the party shows changing images, such as "Again, there are Red Color Alarms," familiar and familiar, a reaction to the abrupt end of the party, but also a feeling of security, as it isn't the first time rockets have been fired. But suddenly, it became apparent that the situation was much broader than rocket fire, as minutes accumulated and another report of terrorists taking control joined the noise of gunfire near, too close.

There's something surreal about a terror attack during a party. The sound of explosions and flashes of light in the sky could easily, at first, seem like an inseparable part of the party, as testified by some of the thousands of participants. You dance all night, with hundreds of people around you, and then comes the dawn. And in Re'im, dawn beside the fields and the surrounding warmth, with rockets flashing above, is not a regular dawn. As the minutes tick by, it's clear that this is a completely different event, one that shouldn't be happening. Around seven o'clock, after the initial alarms, the largest massacre ever to occur in Israel begins, perpetrated by dozens of armed terrorists who arrived at the party, and it doesn't stop for hours. Meanwhile, anyone who can save themselves hides in bomb shelters, in the fields, behind bushes.

Hani's ambulance begins to take in injured people who managed to escape the party. These were injured with a variety of gunshot wounds. One of the girls taken in by the ambulance managed to escape the party. She was hiding inside a bomb shelter with friends and suffered penetrating gunshot wounds in the thigh and shoulder. The two young men sitting beside her were killed. "She bled a lot," says Hani.

She and the paramedic pick up the injured woman, lying on a mattress soaked with blood, on their way to connect her to an intensive care ambulance. Rescue workers gain knowledge of the injury mechanism through the information they see at the scene of the injury, accident, or massacre. With every arrival of an injured person at the hospital, the rescue teams describe the scene itself. This data is collected and documented in the medical file, and this initial aspect is of central importance in all trauma books. When Hani sees an injured woman lying on a mattress soaked with blood, she understands the implication. Generally, shock as a result of bleeding—and in medical terms, "hemorrhagic shock"—is a physiological term that manifests in varying degrees of severity, from mild to severe. Hemorrhagic shock grade 1 means a blood loss not exceeding 15 percent of blood volume, without a significant change in vital signs like pulse or blood pressure. Conversely, hemorrhagic shock grade 4 means a blood loss of over 40 percent of blood volume, or over 2 liters of blood for an adult. This condition is an immediate threat to the patient's life. These are the injured described as in critical condition, they no longer respond to their surroundings, their pulse is extremely high, and their blood pressure is low or even undetectable by a blood pressure monitor. They are at the extreme end of the scale regarding shock as a result of bleeding, and their condition necessitates a rapid blood transfusion.

Therefore, witnessing a field injury with a risk of advanced shock — even if not yet grade 4 — requires an urgent connection to an intensive care ambulance, according to Hani and the paramedic with her. After giving the injured first aid, they contact an intensive care ambulance, transfer her there, and continue their work.

Meanwhile, Avi is in the gathering area, trying to organize aerial evacuation. He is in an area with countless injured soldiers, bodies scattered as if in a war movie, and he is focused on only one thing: triage. Prioritizing who to evacuate first, who would benefit most from rapid evacuation. Alongside the road, a rescue team arrives with a soldier injured by gunfire in the abdomen, semi-conscious, with a rapid pulse and low blood pressure. Next to him lies another soldier with gunshot wounds in the limbs and pelvis. Around, the noise of gunfire, launches, and interceptions can be heard. At the same time, Noemie's ambulance does not stop collecting injured and discharging them, "We simply worked in an endless loop: we loaded injured people in villages, treated them, whether it was to intubate or to stop bleeding and transfer to a helicopter if needed, and then again, back to pick up more injured. I remember one of the injured people I talked to all the way, asking him to hold on, I caressed his head. I told him not to fall asleep."

"You need to understand the courage of the aerial evacuation team. All the time, we have reports around us, it's a war zone, and within record time, we manage to get the injured into the helicopter," Avi recounts. Within four minutes, after intubation and sedation, he and the aerial evacuation team transferred the two soldiers to a helicopter that would take them to the hospital for urgent surgical intervention. The helicopter took off, the skies were clear of clouds but filled with smoke, echoes of explosions, unknown. "We'll be landing with you in a few more minutes," Avi updates the team waiting at the hospital's helipad. On the way, his reserve commander asks him to report in uniform. Avi responds that he is currently on a life-saving mission and will arrive later, and the commander understands. Avi knows that later in the day, he will need to inform his wife that reserve duty is imminent, shortly after gaining control over the infinite number of injured. And he understands that this day is going to be the longest of his life.

Chapter 6: Kidnapped

Barzilai Medical Center in Ashkelon is another southern hospital, smaller than Soroka Medical Center in Be'er Sheva, with about 600 hospital beds. Barzilai provides care for residents of Ashkelon, Sderot, and other southern communities. In recent years, against the backdrop of rocket attacks in the area, the hospital has practiced a structured emergency protocol, in which all hospitalization departments move to the minus two floor in the hospital building, underground. As a pediatric surgeon who occasionally travels there to provide medical care, I have worked several times in this complex, in the underground world of medicine where the usual hospital bustle mixes with the outside alarms and rocket barrages.

This hospital provides a familial atmosphere; almost all its employees live in the Ashkelon area and its surroundings, working for decades in their profession, a fact that speaks to their commitment to their role and a strong loyalty to their workplace, from which you can see the beach of Ashkelon, Delilah Beach.

The blood shed in this region continues from ancient history, to the time when the Philistines — an ancient people who resided in the area until around 600 BCE — were in constant conflict with the Israelites. The most famous stories include Samson the hero, who fought the

Philistines until his death, and his beloved Delilah who betrayed him and revealed the secret of his strength to his enemies. They ruled over five principal and biblical cities: Gath, Gaza, Ashdod, Ashkelon, and Ekron. It is a region adjacent to a beautiful coastline, whose tranquility contrasts with its history as a battleground and site of ongoing conflict, from the days of the patriarchs to our times.

Aliza Lev is a senior social worker at Barzilai Medical Center. It's no coincidence her last name is Lev (Heart in Hebrew). Social work requires a big heart, and a compassionate soul, while dealing with the most difficult moments. When I asked her why she chose this profession, she said she wanted to be exactly at that critical, initial meeting point of a patient who arrives and, besides medical treatment, needs the most basic emotional support. On a daily basis, social workers deal with sad but routine cases that arrive at every hospital's doorstep — abused mothers, neglected children suspected of being abused, road accidents, families without financial support needing social assistance. The vacuum created in these moments of loss, of harsh news, cannot be filled by a doctor or nurse alone. Each has their role in the medical system. The surgeon rushes the patient to surgery, the nurse balances his pain and helps bandage his wounds and feed him, and the social worker connects the puzzle itself, which always arrives scattered in such moments — fragments of life that disintegrated in an instant, needing to be collected and connected to know how to support the child, the mother, the grandmother. A hospital social worker is also skilled in contacting welfare institutions and obtaining various benefits, mediating in crisis moments, coordinating with a psychologist or psychiatrist or other professionals.

Aliza is the social worker responsible for the children's department at Barzilai Medical Center and also works in the large triage room for adult patients. She has been in the role for over 25 years, familiar with all relevant team members, not just medical staff but also, for example, police officers involved in handling complex social cases she deals with. She does about four on-call shifts a month, during which, if there is a crisis event requiring social worker intervention, she goes to the hospital. In our joint work over the past few years, when I meet her, it's always in the wake of a crisis that goes beyond the regular crises of illness, surgery, or hospitalization. Sometimes it involves a baby arriving at the ER with a head injury, and there's suspicion of abuse, requiring the parents to be interviewed as professionally as possible. Occasionally, it's about mediating between former spouses who are no longer in contact. For example, I once encountered a problematic situation involving a father who had cut off all contact with his children and refused urgent surgery for his daughter, and Aliza helped me draft a court petition. In all these cases, I rethink how challenging her role is, facing heartbreaking stories, dealing with broken families, trying to help, and fighting against the slow grinding wheels of justice, if at all. And every time anew, I don't know how her energies never run out, how she doesn't drown.

On 6.10.2023, Friday eve, Aliza was on call. "When I hear the siren of an alarm in Ashkelon, on Saturday around 06:40 in the morning, I realize I need to go to the hospital," she shares. She also lives in Ashkelon, her eldest daughter will later receive a call to report for reserve duty, and her middle daughter is a soldier in the army. Something in Aliza's gut feeling signals to her that although the hospital hasn't yet called her, and although she has already finished her shift, she needs to drive and be present at the ER.

"I arrived at the hospital just before seven. And then suddenly, bodies started arriving," she recounts. By 7:30 a.m., Magen David Adom (MDA) updates that it's a very large mass casualty incident, there are also rumors of many casualties from a party in the Re'im area, and fighting at the Sderot police station, "and suddenly I see that they're bringing in the bodies of police officers from the station in Sderot to the hospital," and it's a scene that's impossible to grasp: a hospital receiving body after body, of police officers in uniform from the station in Sderot, a station she works with.

Aliza recognizes some of them by face, as it's an inherent part of her job, like the work of any social worker in a hospital, mediating between medicine and the regulatory and enforcement systems, for example, between a family known to welfare and a police officer who comes to investigate abuse. And identifying these familiar faces is the first defining moment of an event on a scale that Aliza has never seen before, something she has never experienced, or as she tells me, with her voice cracking, "I realize I know these police officers, from the ongoing work with them. I understand that I suddenly need to separate the fact that I know the names from the fact that I need to function now, and I try to gather myself and not break down."

Many injured people arrive at the ER in large numbers. And the bodies keep coming in an endless stream. Meanwhile, the hospital is also hit by rockets, striking several buildings within the hospital, fortunately without human casualties. Barzilai Medical Center is one of the two hospitals closest to the area currently experiencing a mass casualty event, and throughout the day, it receives hundreds of injured and dozens of dead, and amid all the injured and bodies, Aliza gets a call to go to a family, a mother and three children, one of them severely injured with a serious eye injury. The children themselves are aged ten, twelve, and fifteen. The mother is inconsolable, crying incessantly and receiving sedatives, and the youngest child cries and repeatedly says, "I saw them shoot my father and kill him. Then the terrorist opened the refrigerator door, took out a cola, shot my brother and left."

How do you mediate to a small child the most terrible event on earth? And how do you later tell him that his older brother — the 16-year-old who went to the sea, and everyone was sure he would arrive soon — was also murdered? And where do you even start to breathe? Event follows event, like a movie of horrors, people arrive traumatized, having witnessed horrific acts of slaughter, and suddenly a phone call comes from an anonymous girl named Adi, trapped in a shelter in Be'eri with at least seven bodies on top of her, pleading for rescue. "I don't know what became of her," says Aliza, suddenly silent, "I just kept trying to calm her down, telling her that rescue would come soon, even though I knew I was just buying time. Because the whole area was swarming with terrorists."

In the ER, a mother and her nine-year-old daughter had arrived. The father had been shot in the face and was in critical condition, sedated and intubated, while the mother had collapsed and was in the adult ER, non-communicative and non-functional. The teams were working around the clock, without a moment's rest, but there was a nine-year-old girl now alone in this world, and Aliza took her under her wing. "Her name is Adel," she recounts, "the girl. And I find myself playing the game "City, Country, River" game with her to alleviate her stress, and it's one of the most surreal moments, while we're trying to contact her family to come, but it takes time." What little Adel didn't know was that while Aliza was trying to play with her, she was also managing another event in parallel. Inside Aliza's pocket was the mobile phone of one of the deceased, a phone given to her to keep until the family could be contacted, until they could be informed to come to the hospital.

"I'm playing with Adel, and all the while, I'm preoccupied with thoughts about the dead man's mobile phone in my pocket, constantly waiting for it to ring. It doesn't leave me, and all this time, I feel as if I'm bathing in blood, sensing blood in every corner, and walking around with a lemon in my pocket because the smell won't leave me. For a week, the smell of blood doesn't leave me."

In the midst of the game with little Adel, whom Aliza is looking after until her family can arrive, the mobile phone in her pocket rings. "I take out the mobile phone that just a few hours ago belonged to a living, breathing person," she tries to describe to me how she's pulling out the dead man's phone from her pocket, knowing she has to speak now with family members frantic with worry, and how she tries – even in that moment – to explain to Adel that she's busy for a moment. "I tell the family members to come quickly to Barzilai. We can't deliver the tragic news over the phone, but I will never forget the screams and crying of that day, when the family arrives at the ER and learns the worst."

Together with Aliza is the entire support structure of the hospital, friends and colleagues she has known for years, social workers who encounter horrifying stories, some of whom are simultaneously managing their personal anxiety. One of them is a social worker whose son was at the party in "Re'im," where hundreds of people were slaughtered, and Aliza knows he was at the party, but she has no idea how to mediate the event to her friend. "I see it in her face, as in the faces of everyone who participated in the rescue efforts that day while simultaneously leading a double life in the face of anxiety for family, friends, colleagues. "Simultaneously, I see those who came from the party and were taken to the hospital, and I'm trying to find out where my friend's son is, and if they've heard about him. Only after two days did we find out he was murdered, but at that moment, we were just looking for him in names, in faces, I didn't stop asking about him."

Just then, the realization begins to dawn that it's not only a massacre. There are hostages too. "I'm talking with those who came from the party. They initially thought those moving around in uniforms were soldiers. No one understood at first that these were terrorists opening fire. The terrorists fired as if they were at a shooting range, massively, with the intention to kill, but those survivors from the party suddenly also talk about many people being taken and loaded onto Hamas's trucks and motorcycles, crammed violently and densely, and taken into the Strip."

On Telegram, during those hours, horrifying videos emerge of people loaded onto Hamas's motorcycles and taken into brutal captivity. Israel still believes it's dealing with a few isolated cases of hostages, but reality will slap us in the face when it's revealed, to our utmost horror, that this is one of the largest kidnapping events in history, a mass abduction of women, children and infants, the elderly, and the young.

As we stand before the most terrible nightmare of all.

Chapter 7: Children do not belong in any war

"I was driving to the hospital early in the morning, several alarms had already gone off, and it was obvious something was wrong. I decided to leave the house relatively early. It was at that moment, alone in my office, that I realized the responsibility I have as a pediatrician for the care of Schneider Children's Medical Center's patients." recounts Dr. Efrat Bron-Harlev, Director of Schneider Hospital.

At that moment, when she arrived at the hospital, there was the familiar quiet of a Saturday morning in the hospital, that each medical team member is familiar with in the transition from Friday to Saturday, when only the on-call and duty teams arrive at the hospital, and the usual hustle of a weekday is absent.

Schneider Children's Medical Center is the largest children's hospital in Israel and one of the largest pediatric medical centers in the Middle East. It is located in the center of the country, and comprises hundreds of hospital beds, advanced facilities, and dozens of operating rooms. The vision of its founders, Irving and Helen Schneider, was to build a medical center that would serve as a bridge to peace in the Middle

East. It's important to note that this isn't just a hollow statement, something said to please the medical narrative of making treatment accessible to all who need it. It's a vision filled with substantive action at all levels, including bringing sick children from Gaza, the territories, or other hostile areas to Israel, treating them, including life-saving surgeries, and providing the highest level of medical response.

For example, three years ago, through the mediation of Schneider's contact persons responsible for cooperation between Israel and Gaza, we received a three-year-old boy with a huge tumor in his kidney. It required special cooperation between pediatric surgeons, Cardiothoracic surgeons, anesthetists, invasive angiography teams, oncologists, and intensive care physicians. I remember the day the child and his mother, who accompanied him through all the moments he oscillated between life and death, were discharged back to their home in Gaza, and how all of us were moved by the dramatic life-saving of the little boy, and how many staff members were involved in this extraordinary case.

Dr. Efrat Bron-Harlev has been the director of Schneider Medical Center since 2020. She is a pediatrician with a subspecialty in pediatric intensive care and has been a senior physician in the pediatric intensive care unit at Schneider for years.

Intensive care physicians like Dr. Bron-Harlev, similar to trauma surgeons or doctors working in other acute medical fields, are accustomed to facing death head-on. This profession involves high levels of stress, requiring sharp intuition and quick thinking and action. In other medical fields, we might have the luxury to take our time and make recommendations like, "Follow up in six months at a community clinic," but here, that privilege doesn't exist. When Dr. Harlev wakes up on the morning of October 7th to the sound of consecutive alarms, her gut feeling tells her this is no ordinary event. It's an event that demands a swift journey to the hospital, even before formal reports appear in the news about what's happening under the radar, before we've fully grasped the magnitude of the disaster.

Israel is a country accustomed to the reality of missile attacks and bombings, year after year. I'm not sure that there's another country in the world where children are born into a routine of secure rooms, protected spaces, and knowing how to quickly move to a shelter. While drills for moving to protected spaces or public shelters occur in every significant system worldwide, such as in the United States' education systems, Israel is one of the few places where this threat truly materializes almost every year. And the threat becomes even more complex when it involves a public structure like a large hospital housing hundreds of sick children and their families. When entire hospital departments are not located in protected underground spaces, and a complex and unparalleled transfer operation must begin — involving ventilated patients, preemies weighing half a kilogram, and children connected to ECMO machines. Anywhere else on the globe, moving entire hospital departments on the spot in response to a missile threat on a sovereign nation would likely be detailed on the front pages of the news and described extensively as an unprecedented event. But Israel, as known, is experienced in this matter. Dr. Bron-Harlev remembers the previous event, which was a brief but significant precedent for what unfolded that Saturday.

A year and a half earlier, in May 2021, Hamas launched a massive rocket attack towards Jerusalem and central Israel, involving over 4,000 rockets, missiles, and other bombs. In response, the State of Israel initiated an operation which continued until a ceasefire was achieved, and the rocket threat ceased for that moment. Schneider Medical Center experienced its first experience, in which departments were evacuated to protective zones.

"In 2021, as rockets began to fall massively in the center of Israel, we decided to move all departments to the protected space. There was no other choice. There was a moment, after we had moved all the children to the protected area, where I looked around me and thought to myself, how surreal this was," Dr. Harlev recounts. That day marked a necessary action for her, which lasted ten hours due to the process's complexity but ended successfully. An action designed to ensure the safety of the hospitalized children. "We all believe that children do not belong in any war, that they must be protected. Just as we protect our children at home, so the children in the hospital are like our children."

And here arises the question, how do we, as medical staff, protect children? Moreover, how do we treat them, to what extent are we proactive in our actions?

Shortly after, in 2022, the war between Russia and Ukraine erupted. It was clear to Schneider's management and all teams that the motto according to which children do not belong to any war had to be preserved at all costs. This needed to be done in two main ways: firstly, by bringing sick children from Ukraine to Israel, including providing available medical services for them, and secondly, by establishing a field hospital on Ukrainian soil, with an enhanced team to treat children. Eleven children with various chronic diseases, including kidney failure and cancer, were brought to Israel and to Schneider's departments. The operation to fly them was complex and moving. They were rescued from hell, from a place where they could not survive their chronic illness, and arrived on a night flight to the hospital.

At a conference held later in Europe, attended by managers of children's hospitals from across Europe, Dr. Bron-Harlev spoke about the Israeli experience, the proactive, in bringing sick children from Ukraine to the country. The conference itself coincidentally fell on Holocaust Remembrance Day, which reminded her of the commitment to the other in distress, a commitment that must be expressed actively to bear fruit. The responses were moved, but in some cases, they missed the mark. "I remember a representative from one of the other hospitals noted how happy they would be to receive patients from Ukraine, but it's a pity that the patients from Ukraine haven't arrived yet," she recalls.

The Jewish narrative — the understanding of the importance of active rescue, of the need not to wait but to reach out — took root in the Holocaust of the Jewish people. In other words, rescue cannot be passive, as passivity allowed the Holocaust crime, manifested in the silence of people, communities, and countries while the Nazis' atrocities were committed. At that conference, Dr. Bron-Harlev talked about those children brought to Israel from Ukraine and the new hope for life among those families, and she explained to her colleagues from abroad what would happen if every hospital across Europe was prepared to take in a few children, just like the people who saved another Jewish family and another during World War II, until the State of Israel was established.

The events that occurred just a year and a half ago — as well as the proactivity of Schneider Children's Medical Center, which brought the message of healing to places experiencing severe fighting — remained in Dr. Bron-Harlev's memory. When something stays in our memory, it takes just one gut feeling, like that of a former intensive care physician, to awaken it, to understand that these alarms on a Saturday morning require the exact same approach.

During those hours, like most hospitals in the center of the country, Schneider was flooded with disturbing news about the activation of a mass casualty event and about numerous injured people the likes of which we hadn't known until then. Therefore, it was necessary to work on two fronts simultaneously: to prepare for the possibility that injured children would arrive at Schneider and to move entire departments to a safer place. The alarms continued to sound, and rocket fire did not cease. In addition, many medical staff members began to receive emergency reserve duty orders, whether they were doctors serving as platoon commanders or in operational roles in the military, or doctors serving in various medical roles, including resuscitation teams or rescue teams.

One of these doctors, Dr. Michael Segal, a pediatric surgeon and a close friend of mine from the department, joined his military team and began preparing to head to the south after arming himself and wearing a special vest and continuing with commando unit soldiers to the south.

Dr. Segal had just returned from the United States after participating in a medical conference. That week, he planned to move in with his partner, and the next day, October 8, he was supposed to do a night shift with me in the hospital. But the plans collided with the reality that befell all of us, and he called me that day on his way to the south to update me on the change in plans. Both of us understood, even without words, that he was not going to return to the department soon.

My Boss- the head of the pediatric surgery department at Schneider sent an update to everyone, asking for volunteers to reinforce hospitals in the south if needed, and I found myself writing that I am available for any call. Having just put on her uniform at home, Tamar- my eldest daughter, and her boyfriend, sat with us in front of the TV, unable to take their eyes off the breaking news. Several minutes after receiving the message that I'd been assigned to a reinforcement team at Soroka, Tamar received news from her commanders in the officers' training course that all her classmates were required to report to the train station, likely to be stationed in the south, near the Gaza strip.

I disappeared into the bedroom with red eyes, and she followed me, in uniform, and we both sat on the bed, hugging. And I hadn't cried until now, but everything burst from my eyes.

At the very same hours, many of the hospital staff receive an urgent draft order to the army, amid the noise of alarms. Reports of the injured continue to arrive, and it is clear to everyone that the top priority is to move the hospital departments to a protected area.

"I call the rest of the management team and department heads, and we automatically prepare for the transfer of departments. It is carried out the moment the decision is made, and everyone is there to help," Dr. Bron-Harlev shares. The first to move were the oncology department, children with cancer, who already deal with prolonged hospitalization, difficult treatments, and isolation conditions. The staff of Schneider's Children's Hospital came from home, some without even being called, and did everything they could. Oncology patients being admitted to a new department need everything to be clean, ready for them. They have compromised immune systems; they can't just be transferred carelessly. These are children undergoing extensive chemotherapy protocols, some of whom are in isolation in special rooms, where any exposure to infections could endanger their lives.

Among those participating in this tremendous effort is the Director of Schneider's Emergency Department, Dr. Ron Berant, who arrives with his children from home. "They contributed to the effort, felt they had a part; I didn't see a reason to leave them at home," he says. " It didn't matter what we did—whether it was wiping surfaces with disinfectant wipes, moving equipment, or transferring patients—we provided any help our patients needed."

Dr. Berant, as the director of the country's largest pediatric emergency department, knows to be available all the time. It's an integral part of the profession, ensuring every day that nothing special is happening, that there's no non-routine event, in a place that's always full of non-stop dramas. And that Saturday grips him by the throat and does not let go, of him and his children. Dr. Berant accompanies his children during the transition of the oncology department and the intensive care unit. His daughter, who completed a medics course in

Magen David Adom, walks with an Ambu bag giving oxygen to one of the babies, along with countless other team members, including doctors, nurses, support staff, and volunteers.

Dr. Efrat Bron-Harlev is leading this massive effort—moving entire departments, with children connected to breathing machines, one after the other, to protected spaces- and when there are moments of anxiety, like when someone reports on another horrifying and unbelievable video, when someone says it's not just a few terrorists, it's hundreds, thousands, when Dr. Berant's son receives a message from a friend and gets anxious, saying, "Dad, they say there are terrorists roaming the country," just at the moment they are moving another patient, Dr. Berant says to his son, "listen now, there are no terrorists. Now there's only the child in front of us. He needs us, and that's it." And his son resets himself and returns to function.

And in those morning hours, when Dr. Bron-Harlev's gut feeling signals to her that this is not a normal event, Dr. Amit Frenkel, an intensive care physician and the doctor responsible for mass casualty events at Soroka in times of emergency, understands that he is about to declare a mass casualty event in advance. He just doesn't yet know that it will be the largest mass casualty event in the history of the State of Israel, and one of the largest in the entire world.

Chapter 8: Game changer

Dr. Amit Frenkel is an intensive care physician at Soroka Hospital. He is married and a father of three, his wife is a psychiatrist, and his eldest son is a soldier serving in the south of the country. The family lives in Meitar, a small pastoral settlement a fifteen-minute drive from Soroka. In times of emergency at the hospital, Dr. Frenkel takes on a different role: managing mass casualty events.

In every mass casualty event, logistical preparation is of immense importance. Few deal with it as the injured arrive, but it must be considered in advance, and even while in motion. The first step is the very declaration of a mass casualty event. Who declares such an event, and what does it mean for the hospital? Declaring a mass casualty event is a formal act. It is usually done by the hospital director and requires special steps that go beyond the hospital's routine. Similar to a country declaring war, declaring a mass casualty event means that the hospital urgently summons teams from home, and simultaneously transforms various sites to prepare for the admission of the injured.

It's a moment that deviates from any other event in any hospital worldwide, because it's the main event for so many patients and staff members. It's a declaration that transforms the hospital into a different place. Anyone who has never seen an ER prepare to a mass casualty event will be amazed at the immense logistical operation that arises out of nowhere, with doctors, nurses, para-medical teams, and logistics personnel arriving in droves, wearing special vests reserved only for these events. The blood bank enters a state of exceptional readiness for a massive blood transfusions, the ER is cleared within a short time to make room for the injured, whole departments discharge patients to their homes or other hospitals, all to enable treatment for dozens, perhaps even hundreds, of injured people.

On that Saturday morning, Dr. Frenkel is awakened by the sound of explosions. He understands that these are rockets coming from the Gaza Strip. Within a few minutes, he receives a message from his son in the army, in the south area. His son updates Dr. Frenkel that there was a red alert and that he and the other soldiers are protected in a shelter. Given the unusual number of alerts across the country and bits of information received on social networks, he decides to head to the hospital, where the hospital's senior management also arrives.

Soroka Hospital employs over 5,000 staff members, many of whom live in southern towns, including those close to the border of the Gaza strip. Messages from employees in areas where terrorists have infiltrated paint a horrifying picture, indicating a high potential for a mass casualty event, even in the early hours before a large number of injured would justify initiating a mass casualty protocol.

Dr. Amit Frenkel, deciding along with the hospital's management to activate the mass casualty protocol ahead of time before many injured had arrived at the hospital, described the decision as a life-saving game-changer. The early mobilization of staff, as well as keeping the night shift teams at the hospital, allowed for early preparation for the event.

The change of shifts at 07: 00 AM in most hospitals is a time when the night team hands over to the morning team, with nurses conducting an orderly shift change in all departments, and doctors ending their shifts and reporting to the incoming doctor on duty. The decision to keep the night staff at the hospital, along with the activation of the mass casualty protocol, led to over a thousand employees being present at the hospital shortly after the event began.

Dr. Frenkel wasn't the only one arriving at those moments of uncertainty and many questions. Dr. Eitan Neeman, who was on call that weekend and intended to complete a visit, arrived at the pediatric intensive care unit. Weekend on-call doctors arrive in the morning, like on a regular workday, and stay as long as needed, with work in intensive care often not ending at a specific time. But on October 7, the hospital quickly filled with injured patients. Dr. Neeman positioned himself in the trauma room to assist in treating injured children. Shortly after, he received an urgent call and was requested to join his military reserve unit. The head of the pediatric intensive care unit arrived from home, took over for Dr. Neeman in the trauma room, and Dr. Neeman left for the military gathering point.

Dr. Frenkel and his colleagues remember the dedicated and cheerful doctor parting from them to head into a dire situation, as they were in the midst of a war that manifested not only in critically injured patients being evacuated but also in massive rocket fire threatening the hospital.

"One have to understand the problematic situation in which we must manage a mass casualty event, while simultaneously facing ceaseless alarms and rockets firing near the hospital itself," adds Dr. Frenkel. "If in any other mass casualty event the hospital remains outside the conflict zone, here we faced two issues: an increasingly massive intake of injured, and red alert alarms that required staff protection. Unfortunately, there are areas in the hospital that are not protected, including some of the operating rooms. The staff who were outside the hospital handling the initial triage of the injured had to enter a protected area with the injured at every alarm. This naturally created difficulty in initial sorting."

By 09:00 AM, hundreds of doctors, nurses, and other staff members gathered in Soroka's emergency room, starting to treat the injured who were arriving. The rate of injured arriving increased – dozens per hour from different locations, including soldiers, civilians, and attendees of the Nova festival in Kibbutz Re'im. Some arrived independently, by car. Some were evacuated by ambulances, and helicopters began to land one after another. Dr. Frenkel was responsible for managing this massive operation, including control over the emergency room and treating everyone. In the afternoon, the peak rate of injured arrivals occurred, with a record number of over 80 injured entering the hospital within the most intensive hour and more than 680 injured patients throughout the day, including over 130 in critical condition.

Several sites in any hospital are crucial for managing a mass casualty event. One is the emergency room. During a mass casualty event, the emergency room becomes entirely different, emptied of all "regular" patients who quickly ascend to inpatient departments, turning into an intake site for injured patients and those arriving with symptoms of anxiety.

Each type of injury has a dedicated team waiting with sheets and sequential numbers. Amid this, in addition to doctors and nurses, social workers, psychologists, and psychiatrists rush to support all those with anxiety and shock, all patients who witnessed horrors and are struggling to speak and function. Other critical sites include the operating rooms prepared to accept injured for emergency surgeries.
But perhaps the most critical site, in terms of managing the injured, is the shock room or trauma room. Adjacent to the emergency room, it typically looks like a small hall with several beds, each fully equipped with a ventilator, sets for treating severely injured patients, a monitor, and life-saving equipment. From here, after initial stabilization, the most critical patients are moved to one of three key locations: an operating room, a CT scan, or intensive care unit.

Next to each bed in the shock room, an average of five or six team members are treating a severely injured patient. One is the patient care manager, usually the most senior doctor on the team, skilled in trauma management. This doctor is primarily responsible for the patient and determines the treatment order. Another doctor is positioned at the patient's head, responsible for the airway, performing sedation and ventilation as needed. Simultaneously, another doctor conducts a rapid examination of the injured and also manages life-saving procedures. Additionally, at least three nurses are responsible for undressing the patient, taking vital signs, administering fluids, blood, and medications. Just one patient in the shock room can give it an appearance of constant hustle and bustle. Soroka has six such beds, prepared to handle six patients simultaneously, but it quickly becomes evident that even this is not sufficient.

Dr. Frenkel and his colleagues realize that the influx of patients, many of whom are in a critical or even life-threatening condition, necessitates doubling the capacities in the trauma room. "We add six more beds to the trauma room, reaching a situation where we are treating 12 injured individuals at any given time," he explains. This decision was significant and helped the hospital cope with the event. "At times, we had about a hundred staff members in the trauma room, with more and more injured arriving, many of whom were then moved to surgery or intensive care," he notes.

In all the chaos, he tries to contact his son, the soldier, in the few seconds he can spare, because personal issues cannot be entirely set aside, and in all the unimaginable moments of that Saturday morning, personal and professional lives intertwine. Dr. Frenkel's son does not respond for many, too many, hours. And it's not just Dr. Frenkel who experiences this, but also one of the nurses in the emergency room, whose son was called up for emergency military service and went to the front. She tries to function automatically and not think about the dangers.

Rotem, the nurse, who is deep into her work at Sheba Medical Center, where the injured from the south are being brought in rapid evacuation and ambulances, experiences similar feelings. Hospitals in the central region were updated about the mass casualty event declared at Soroka and Barzilai, and many staff members are also heading to hospitals in the central region to help with the intake of injured. Rotem dashes between intensive care and the emergency area, preparing the ground for rapid intake, but her heart is anxious for her family, and in the family WhatsApp group, she waits for a response from Shira, her niece, who is in Nahal Oz, close to the Gaza Strip border.

"Shira writes to all of us in the family WhatsApp group that she is in the war room, that they are okay," Rotem notes. It was around 9:30 AM, and Rotem is just about to prepare the new intensive care beds at Sheba, which were supposed to open in a month, but the terrorist attack brought their early use. Shortly after Shira, Rotem's niece, updates her family that she is okay, Dr. Frenkel's son also updates that he is in a bunker somewhere, safe. Both Rotem and Amit take a brief moment to breathe a sigh of relief and get back to work.

Among all these places in Soroka – the trauma room, the emergency room, the operating rooms – Iris Raz, the nurse, and Dr. Yael Levaot, responsible for the hospital's resilience framework, rush about. Early on, they understand that many staff members are trapped in communities threatened by terrorists, and they recognize the need to contact them, check on their well-being, and determine how to evacuate them. They quickly compile a list of all staff members living in danger areas and begin to make contact. Some staff members do not answer, some whisper they are under attack, that there are terrorists in their community. They manage to contact Dr. Daniel Levy, an ENT doctor from Soroka who is in a clinic in Kibbutz Be'eri, treating injured under terrorist attack from outside. He tells them there is a dead and injured person, he has no way to protect himself, and asks them to call for help. They contact the police, which promises to do its best, and there's still hope in the air that rescue is coming. Then Iris receives a phone call from her husband, who is in the Southern

Command's operations center. "Iris, I need your help," he says, "You need to be strong for what I'm about to tell you." He's not usually so grave, she notices. She's prepared.

"There's a woman, in her ninth month of pregnancy, from Kibbutz Be'eri, in severe labor pains, trapped in a safe room, who managed to contact the command center," her husband tells her. "Do you know a midwife in the area who could help her?"

Chapter 9: They also shoot pregnant women

"I'm calling Adrian," Iris recounts. It's noon, and Iris has just ended the call with her husband who relayed distressing news from his command center: an unidentified pregnant woman is trapped in a safe room in Kibbutz Be'eri, with no way to reach her. Iris, who worked for years as a midwife before moving into administrative roles, knows exactly who to turn to first—Adrian, the legendary midwife of Soroka Hospital, who resides in the very kibbutz where the woman with severe labor pains is reported to be. Adrian is retired but her experience is vast. She came to Israel at a young age for a brief visit, fell in love with the south, particularly the kibbutz, and stayed forever. Until her retirement, she worked as a midwife at Soroka Hospital, delivering thousands of women.

The tension in the command center is mounting with harsh reports of battles with terrorists and people pleading for help. Iris tries calling Adrian several times to no avail. She can't reach her by any means and suspects that Adrian too is trapped under the terrorists' control. Deciding to seek help elsewhere, she turns to a physiotherapist she knows from Soroka, who also lives in Kibbutz Be'eri. The childbirth pains, which should be an exciting if painful backdrop to the arrival of new life, become in her imagination a chilling nightmare she can't shake off.

Meanwhile, Prof. Eyal Sheiner, a gynecologist and the head of the Obstetrics and Gynecology Department, also arrives at Soroka. Living in Omer, near Be'er Sheva, he wakes up to the sound of alarms, like everyone else. One of the department's first challenges at that moment is the transition to protected structures. The hospital is under relentless missile attack from Gaza, and not all buildings are fortified, including the gynecology departments themselves. The teams start organizing and moving, but suddenly, there's a report of another pregnant woman, due to give birth soon, who was shot in the abdomen—a report that catches Prof. Sheiner's team amid preparations for relocation.

Among all the complex trauma cases, the trauma of a pregnant woman is considered one of the most complex to treat—emotionally, physiologically, and systematically—requiring the involvement of several different teams.

As doctors, we aim to care for two patients intertwined: the mother and the fetus. The mother, like any pregnant woman, presents unique physiological aspects that a trauma specialist must recognize. For instance, the expanding uterus presses on the venous return and the inferior vena cava, potentially leading to decreased cardiac output. The abdominal organs themselves shift: the stomach is pushed upward, and the intestines are pushed aside to make room for the growing fetus within the uterus. On the other hand, we're aware of the complexity of treating the fetus, which only near birth matures its systems, including the brain, heart, lungs, kidneys, and intestines, preparing for extracorporeal life where all systems can function after leaving the womb.

Among all complex trauma types—blunt injury, sharp object injury, or gunshot wound—a gunshot wound is one of the most complicated. It's impossible to predict the trajectory of a bullet fired into the body. A shot from a handgun differs from a sniper rifle, for example. The bullet's speed, size, and shape determine the extent of damage to body tissues, and almost nothing can be predicted in advance. For instance, the entry wound doesn't indicate where the exit wound, if any, will be. Combining these two types of injuries—a pregnant woman with a penetrating gunshot wound—escalates the complexity.

In other words, a fetus in a pregnant woman's womb presents a physiological challenge, as does the pregnant woman herself. Each of these entities is a whole, and between them exists a marvelous symbiotic system. However, when it comes to life-and-death situations, there's one crucial principle learned in trauma lessons across various medical units: the best treatment for the fetus begins with ensuring the mother is well treated. This is because the fetus will exhibit distress the moment it senses its mother is losing blood, entering shock, or deteriorating due to a severe infectious process. Therefore, contrary to maternal instinct, which prioritizes the child's well-being above one's own, the approach here is similar to the emergency instructions on passenger planes, where an adult is shown putting on an oxygen mask first before helping their child—first, care for the mother, then for the baby.

Professor Sheiner arrives at the trauma room where a woman in her ninth month of pregnancy is located. The initial report is of shrapnel injury to the abdomen—like any trauma patient, the first concern is the vital signs of the mother—blood pressure, pulse, and oxygen saturation measurement. While caring for the mother herself and assessing her hemodynamic stability, there is a simultaneous assessment of the fetus—an ultrasound scan shows that the fetus is viable, with a normal heartbeat and a normal amount of amniotic fluid. Despite these initially good findings, evidence of a gunshot wound dictates a rapid and even immediate response—it's impossible to overlook the small entry wound into the pregnant woman's abdomen, and urgent surgery is necessary. The woman's husband reports that she was shot directly in the abdomen, and Professor Sheiner cannot contain his horror.

They also shoot pregnant women.

The mother is quickly transferred to the operating room, where she is stable. The plan is for emergency surgery and the rescue of the fetus, assessing whether there are additional injuries in the mother's abdominal cavity due to the penetrating gunshot wound, and hoping with a heavy heart that both mother and fetus will survive. Upon entering the abdominal cavity in the operating room, the gynecologists identify the entry hole of the bullet penetration in the uterus. They immediately rescue the little fetus straight to the pediatric medical team, which is ready to receive her and assess her condition. Unfortunately, it turns out that the fetus is injured—the pediatrician identifies an entry and exit wound in her lower abdomen, and urgent intervention of a pediatric surgeon is needed.

"I think I drove at 200 kilometers per hour to the hospital that day, already that morning, and even before we were called to the operating room," Dr. Zaki Asi, head of the pediatric surgery department at Soroka, recounts. Dr. Asi is an expert in pediatric surgery and general surgery. He began his career in general surgery, and after completing his residency in general surgery, he decided to further specialize in pediatric surgery. Working in the field of pediatric surgery requires a unique understanding of a wide range of patients. It is fundamentally different from general surgery in adults, not only because of the different and unique pathologies in children but also—primarily—because of the wide variety of patients.

On an average day, a pediatric surgeon might operate on a preemie weighing just a few hundred grams in the morning, treat a one-year-old baby next, and then operate on a fifteen-year-old teen. At every age, there are nuances and different physiologies. As a pediatric surgeon, I realized that this is one of the most heterogeneous professions out there during one of my shifts, where I ran to an emergency surgery for a critically ill preemie weighing five hundred grams, and after that, I operated on a girl with appendicitis who was almost 18 years old. A teen is not a child, and a child is not a baby, and a preemie is utterly different from all of these—in its fragility, its ability to survive, its scant reserves.

The greatest complexity lies with the fetus emerging into new life. At the miraculous moment of a baby's birth, immense physiological changes occur where the fetus begins to breathe for the first time. The small lungs, which until that moment during pregnancy were underdeveloped and almost didn't require blood supply, start to function, and the first breaths inflate the lungs, which then receive a significant blood supply. Concurrently, the fetal circulation converts to adult circulation, and the cutting of the umbilical cord is just one part in a series of marvelous steps at the end of which the baby becomes a physiologically independent entity.

Even a minor injury to this delicate mechanism—such as a fetus injured while still in its mother's womb—can be fatal.

Dr. Asi receives a report about a pregnant woman undergoing emergency surgery suffering from a penetrating gunshot wound, and the pediatric surgery team steps in, preparing an operating room for a newborn who has yet to take her first breath of new life. "We see that she has a bullet lodged in the abdominal wall, and another that penetrated towards the pelvis, with a rear exit hole. There was a need to surgically explore the pelvic area."

Anyone not involved in pediatric surgery and hearing Dr. Asi's description might not fully understand the level of delicacy and caution required in operating on such a small infant. "The bleeding vessels in the pelvis of a newborn are as tiny as she is, and the surgical challenge combined with the fact that the baby has just been born raises fears she won't survive," he notes. Additionally, the coagulation functions of a newborn and the ability to overcome penetrating injuries—even after a successful surgery—are not sufficiently developed. One of the first things done in every nursery around the world, for example, is administering vitamin K to the baby a few hours after birth, because newborns are born with low levels of this vitamin, essential for proper blood clotting in the body and for the production of clotting factors in the liver. Despite the team's efforts to

90

compensate for all deficiencies, there's a significant concern for her life. Yet, at this stage, the surgery is nearing completion, and the hope is that the bleeding has stopped and that the injuries were repaired during the surgery. The little baby is transferred to the neonatal intensive care unit, in serious but stable condition.

After Dr. Asi completes surgery on a child whose father was murdered in a brutal attack, suffering from a gunshot wound across the abdomen with holes in the intestines, spleen, and diaphragm, amid hours filled with additional surgeries he participates in, he receives an update that the operated baby girl is unstable and enters a vicious cycle- the baby enters a process of disseminated intravascular coagulation (DIC), a destructive process where clotting factors in the body are excessively activated, creating numerous blood clots that sweep along platelets and cause a shortage of platelets.

The outcome can be fatal, involving extensive bleeding that is nearly impossible to stop, combined with blood clots that affect blood supply to the tissues. Surgeons refer to this process as non-surgical bleeding, meaning there is no good way to stop it, as it doesn't involve a single blood vessel that can be tied or cauterized. It concerns a patient who bleeds from every touch, unable to maintain the delicate and unique clotting process. When there's no good way to stop such bleeding, all that remains is to pray.

The medical teams' prayers join those of countless families crowding the emergency room, trying in vain to locate their loved ones among the multitude of injured patients, many of whom are still unidentified. Heart-wrenching cries echo in the corridors, where people walk with large signs of their missing family members' photos since the morning hours. Hospital teams try to organize and rapidly identify all patients, whether through photos taken even in the operating room or through a data registry set up from scratch. Meanwhile, events that defy imagination occur, redefining what human drama is, such as the small fetus who ultimately couldn't survive the gunshot wound, or the pregnant woman in a kibbutz who was trapped in a secure room in labor pains and was murdered alongside her fetus found lying next to her.

As the medical staff treat the wounded, they receive urgent reserve duty calls. There's no time to absorb the meaning, though it's clear to everyone: The State of Israel has entered a war.

Chapter 10: Golden hour

Dr. A is a physician in an elite unit in the army. The Medical Corps is a unique branch in the Israel Defense Forces. It consists of a medical team whose mission is to save lives and not to actively engage in warfare on one hand, but on the other hand, they must be skilled in using weapons. The role is dual: to assist, protect, and treat, but at the same time, to be operationally fit as a fighter. Within the military framework, doctors and medical personnel such as paramedics and medics serve in a variety of roles, ranging from combat soldiers who transitioned to become medics, through army medics who completed a one-year course within the military framework, to doctors, some of whom serve in regular army service that they began during their pre-military education, and some are doctors who reinforce the ranks during reserve duty.

Being a physician in an elite unit requires high operational readiness. These are doctors who are in top units and closely accompany the fighters in conditions that can be harsh, threatened by the enemy, conditions that require adaptation to field conditions, and a rapid understanding of the world of trauma and treatment of the wounded under suboptimal conditions.

Dr. A is married and a father of three. "On that Saturday morning, I came to the hospital for a shift" he tells me. "I am a resident in general surgery, but I'm also serve as a doctor in an elite unit in the army, and at around seven o'clock in the morning, after I arrive at the department and prepare to take over the department, they call me from my unit and tell me to come urgently."

Dr. A leaves the hospital, comes home, and tells his wife that they'll probably inform him any moment that he doesn't need to come, and he'll return to the hospital, but in his heart, he already has a feeling of war. Within minutes, he leaves with full gear towards the unit where he serves as a physician. In our conversation, he recalls that on the way to the unit, he saw a huge column of smoke rising from somewhere, presumably from the explosion of a rocket in the area.

"Just a few minutes after I arrived at the unit and we received our equipment, including weapons, we get on a vehicle, leave the unit a little before nine in the morning, and receive our first mission. In the same vehicle, there are no other doctors or medics with me, and I understand that the responsibility for treating the wounded is on me. On the way, we are updated about a change in mission. Our mission is to reach Kibbutz Be'eri. There is an update that there are infiltrators in the surrounding settlements, and we need to go and extract the wounded."

A's mother lives in Kibbutz Nir Oz, a kibbutz also located in the surrounding area. Dr. A calls her on the way, after the team was informed about the infiltration of terrorists. "As far as I'm concerned, this was my last conversation with my mother," he tells me, "She whispers to me that there are terrorists in her kibbutz and that she can't talk anymore, and I leave for the mission in Kibbutz Be'eri with a deep fear that I won't speak to her anymore. That she won't survive this day."

Dr. A still doesn't know the extent of the situation. He just understands that it's something very significant, fundamentally different from any event he has ever participated in. "We understand fairly quickly that the main road, Route 232, is threatened by terrorists, and we consider ways to reach Kibbutz Be'eri, but the vehicle is stopped due to gunfire, and we are forced to dismount, meaning, to start walking with all our equipment, when shortly after another vehicle from the unit joins us to reinforce us, and then finally, another medic from the unit joins me.

"We plan to reach Kibbutz Be'eri via off-road routes, through areas like Shokeda Forest, where I've traveled with the kids to the Red South Festival. And it's October and there's no anemone bloom, the entire expanses of the Red South are empty, and it's a strange, surreal feeling," Dr. A notes as they realize in the background that there's no choice but to cross the main road towards the kibbutz.

Along the way, they encounter several incidents, including heavy gunfire, ambushes, RPG missiles. "We establish phone contact with the kibbutz's deputy security officer, plan to pass through a water crossing, or from the logistic area — just not from the main gate, which is threatened and controlled by terrorists."

During those hours, Kibbutz Be'eri is filled with hundreds of terrorists who occupy the kibbutz, going from house to house, attempting to break into homes and capture people inside. Like in any kibbutz, one of the central buildings is the kibbutz clinic, the place that on a daily basis is the first point of contact for medical assistance. Amit Mann, a paramedic with Magen David Adom (MDA), who worked at Kibbutz Be'eri as a paramedic, left her residential unit in the kibbutz towards the dental clinic after initial reports arrived about terrorists infiltrating the kibbutz and injured arriving — one in critical condition — at the clinic itself. Some people choose to be paramedics because it sounds challenging and inspiring to them, some because this profession means there's never a dull moment on the side, and some, like Amit, seem to have been born for it. Born to heal.

"We're five sisters, Amit was the youngest, really the baby of the family," recounts Haviva Mann, Amit's sister. "When Amit was born, I was already 17, and we always doted on her, who would bathe her, who would dress her, who would watch over her. She was our princess, the youngest of four older sisters." The family lives in Netivot, five daughters, a mom, and a dad. "Our dad was diagnosed with advanced cancer when Amit was ten years old, and she was very attached to him, he was an amazing father, and for four years he fought the disease. and Amit understood what she wanted to be when she grew up — a doctor."

During the years when doctors and nurses came and went and supported their father, Amit saw how they eased his suffering, and she called them angels in white.

"At the age of 15, she volunteered for Magen David Adom (MDA), but it was much more than just volunteering. She would go after school to the library, read medical books, copy body systems, and draw everything she learned on sheets. When I came back on leave from the army, I had to test her on all sorts of medical questions she asked," says Haviva, "and in parallel with the first aid course and the paramedic course, she did so much more. She had an amazing voice, she sang all the time, performed in musicals, her charm was irresistible. And always with amazing humility, as if she didn't hold so many talents, as if she wasn't blessed with amazing vocal abilities, with talent for acting, with a love for people that amazed us every time anew."

At the age of 18 and a half, Amit graduated with honors from the paramedic course and began saving lives. She planned to study medicine later and meanwhile fulfilled dream after dream. She was always the first to arrive at accident and bombing scenes, and she always took every case as a mission, made sure to stay in touch with patients she met during her shift, visited hospitals, went to comfort mourners in their home. "Every patient for her was a world unto themselves. The moment she loved most was when they called her for a birth. For a woman in labor, attacked at the checkpoints and who called for an ambulance, it was a moment of pure joy for her. She radiated happiness and shared these moments with us all the time."

A year and a half before October 2023, Amit started working as a trained paramedic at Kibbutz Be'eri, in addition to her work at MDA. Every kibbutz has a small clinic open until afternoon hours and closed thereafter, including on weekends and holidays. A trained paramedic is a medical team member who provides assistance during hours when the clinic is closed and is responsible for shifts during the week and weekends. "She was happy- she had her own living unit, and she did exactly what she wanted to do, and she progressed to become the lead instructor in MDA's paramedic course in the Southern District, the youngest lead instructor in the country. And despite the intensive work, the training, and the lifesaving, she continued to sing. It was her therapy, entering her room in our home in Netivot and singing with a deep, clear, beautiful voice, and it was clear to us that she could have been a star to the same extent, but she preferred the world of medicine," Haviva told me.

On the day before October 7th, the family WhatsApp group was filled with moments just before the holiday. One of the sisters in Be'er Sheva tried to persuade Amit to postpone her duty in Be'eri for another time and come to eat a family meal with them, and Amit responded that she allows herself to keep the invitation for another time, and the sun set and rose again for the last time, on Amit, on Saturday morning.

"We all started messaging the moment the missiles started, and Amit packed her bag, put on her gear, and hurried to the clinic, even though her partner, who stayed with her that night, is also a paramedic by profession, tried to persuade her to leave the kibbutz because it's dangerous. She answered him, precisely because it's dangerous, that's why I need to stay here, and she stayed at the clinic."

In the early hours, when the terrorists' attack on the kibbutz began, Amit called for help incessantly and requested that an ambulance arrive, and in the meantime, she provided medical treatment together with Dr. Daniel Levi, who ran, also, to the dental clinic, and the kibbutz nurse, Nirith, who felt the need to help. The clinic team included two trained individuals, equipped with rifles, who tried their best to defend the wounded who arrived at the clinic, facing dozens of terrorists who started going from house to house and marked the clinic as a target for occupation. The team managed to provide medical treatment to at least five or six injured people, and even when the medical supplies ran out, Amit tried to encourage the wounded, provide compassion and humanity, and provide telephone assistance to the kibbutz residents who pleaded for help from their fortified homes.

"We're talking about a 22-year-old girl with a strong spirit and professionalism who continued to be connected to the kibbutz WhatsApp group and tried to help, even though the situation was dire and the terrorists were about to take over the clinic. She chose to stay and help the wounded even though she could have stayed in the safe room in her apartment and protected herself. She remained true to herself," her sister said. Reading the family conversations fills me with waves of deep sorrow. The conversations describe moments of realization that this is the end, and moments of helplessness that stretch to the edge of Amit's family, who are unable to help. And when her beloved sister calls, she only hears with horror the last words of her younger sister, "They shot me in the leg," she responds when the terrorists burst into the clinic and almost killed everyone there, "They're on me," she adds, and the call disconnects, and darkness descends on the last conversation. And at those very moments, as Amit struggles in her final moments while trying to save lives in the clinic in Be'eri, Dr. A. struggles to reach the kibbutz.

The arrival at the kibbutz, after all the changes along the way and the encounters, only occurs in the afternoon, around 12:30. In retrospect, it turned out that more than hundred of terrorists had entered the kibbutz and they controlled the main traffic routes. "When I arrive, there are already wounded people, and we decide to treat all the injured in a secure place together with the military, and with additional medics and fighters who secured us, while the rest of the force continues further into the depths of the kibbutz to fight the terrorists and save as many civilians as possible."

The first casualty they treated, Dr. A explains to me, suffered a significant cervical injury as a result of severe neck wounds. The neck is one of the critical areas in penetrating trauma. It is an exposed area, relatively, where major blood vessels—the carotid artery and the jugular vein—run on both sides, as well as the airway (trachea) in its center, so penetrating injuries can be lethal. One reason is a major bleeding from blood vessel, and another reason is injured airway.

"We managed to stabilize this casualty, give him plasma and painkillers, and successfully evacuate him, when shortly thereafter another fighter arrived with a critical gunshot wound, requiring the insertion of two chest tubes and securing the airway by performing a cricothyroidotomy. This casualty is in a critical condition and loses vital signs in a matter of minutes on the scene, despite the rapid attempt to control his severe injuries."

At this point, Dr. A realizes that he is in a situation where soldiers from his unit are being killed beside him, people he has known for years. Friends. The next casualty arrives with a gunshot wound to the hip, there is a huge hole in the right thigh, he is pale and combative, trying to resist treatment, "and I realize that this is a 'C' casualty, but that if he is not evacuated immediately, he will die."

The Golden Hour in trauma care is a well-known term in the treatment of trauma casualties of all kinds. Generally, from an epidemiological perspective, the death of trauma casualties is distributed into three points on the timeline. At the first point on the timeline are casualties who die within seconds or a few minutes of the event. These are critical casualties suffering from devastating head injuries, injuries involving major blood vessels, etc. The chance of saving them in the field is close to zero.

At the second point are casualties who die within a few hours. These are treated casualties suffering from injuries or severe trauma, such as ruptured spleen, pneumothorax, or significant damage to vital organs. This is where the definition of the ″Golden Hour″ comes in, meaning that if we, as caregivers, manage to identify and treat the casualties within an hour, giving them blood products, performing an urgent chest decompression, controlling bleeding—we can save them.

At the third point on the timeline of trauma casualty mortality are casualties who die days to weeks after the injury. Death in these cases usually occurs among hospitalized casualties with severe injuries, who die from various complications, such as infections, organ failure, etc.

The idea of the ″Golden Hour″ is intended to help the medical staff quickly identify life-threatening injuries, those that can be identified and treated within minutes. To help the staff identify these injuries quickly, a trauma treatment model called ATLS (Advanced Trauma Life Support) was developed. Every surgeon in the world is required to be familiar with the principles of the model, which include several simple rules. The main one is to identify the most life-threatening injury of all, to treat it, and to move on to the next priority. For this purpose, injuries are classified according to severity. The most severe injury in terms of medical urgency is the loss of the airway, marked with an A. The moment the patient is injured in the area related to the airway, or if his level of consciousness drops so much that he is unable to maintain the airway, he will not survive because he cannot breathe. Therefore, this is the first priority in treating any trauma casualty.

The second most severe injury is in the respiratory system- breathing, hence marked with a B. This is a casualty with no injury to their airway, but they are unable to oxygenate themselves effectively due to various reasons, as their lungs are damaged, chest cavity is compromised, etc. Such a casualty will also not survive, as they will not be able to breathe effectively. The next system in importance is circulation, marked with a C, and therefore it is important to check if the patient is losing blood or fluids and is at risk of developing hypovolemic shock.

When Dr. A sees the soldier next to him bleeding into his pelvis, and he is busy changing bandages and applying direct pressure to the bleeding area, he begins to realize two things: One, that injuries with compromised circulation and acute bleeding are about to become the main injuries. The second thing he understands at that moment is that his plasma and equipment in the field are running out. This happens just before A's unit manages to evacuate the bleeding soldier from the kibbutz, and they decide to head towards the main emergency road which was already secured at this stage- but this is not the end, this is hardly the beginning. "we suddenly see huge masses of casualties that arrive. From everywhere. They come by ambulance, in cars, from all sorts of places, a crazy number of casualties."

South of Kibbutz Be'eri, near the border, lies the kerem Shalom base. It is one of the southernmost bases closest to the border with Egypt and the border with the Gaza Strip. Normally, Noam Barel serves there as a paramedic in the IDF. The IDF paramedics course is one of the prestigious and lengthy courses available. It lasts a year and two months, during which the soldier commits to serving almost two additional years in mandatory service. The training also includes internships in hospitals, volunteering with Magen David Adom during leaves for standby duties, and providing medical assistance to civilians and soldiers. Noam is a certified paramedic, serving at the Kerem Shalom base with her team. Every nine days, they go home for five days of vacation. That particular Saturday, she was at the Kerem Shalom base, on a reduced medical staff setup, meaning one less medic than usual.

"We're getting Red Alert sirens and booms as a result of rockets hitting the base, and then we all rush to the bomb shelter," she tells me, adding that she always wanted to be a paramedic, volunteering for Magen David Adom since the age of 15, and it was clear she would continue in the army. "Several soldiers from various units, cooks, and fighters also come to our shelter, and after about half an hour, we suddenly hear a base announcement that terrorists have infiltrated."

Noam and the other soldiers in the shelter were very skeptical at this point about reports of terrorist infiltration. The concept was that even if a terrorist penetrated the fence from Gaza, he would not be able to cross the base's main security line. But very quickly, they realized this was a different event. "We heard a lot of gunfire. The shelter was open, without a door, so we hid inside. There was no choice, and we kept all the phones on silent," she recalls. At some point, she decided to peek outside and see what was happening, and the scene was unbelievable: terrorists roaming the base, dressed in black with green headbands. "I couldn't even text my parents, there wasn't much reception either, we're just trying to understand what's happening at any given moment and stay quiet so they don't find us."

Noam, like Dr. A, quickly found herself in an almost impossible situation, setting up a field treatment point under threat, while her medical resources were dwindling rapidly, and she faced many casualties and severe injuries requiring blood products.

With the terrorists' infiltration, combat began at the base. Another medical team updated her that she had to go to the area where they were treating the wounded, which was on the other side of the base, as there were many casualties. Under the cover of armed soldiers, she hurried to another shelter, and there she and the military paramedic in the second team began treating the wounded who were brought to the area without interruption. "The ambulance of the second medical team was burned at the base as a result of a rocket fired at it, so the only medical equipment was in my ambulance, which was far away, and the fighters at the base risked gunfire to bring medical supplies to us all the time. There was a stage where there were only two units of plasma left but more casualties, and it was necessary to decide who was more urgent for treatment."

In the midst of managing the treatment of the wounded, as the scale of the event became apparent to Noam, she realized she had to update her family that she was okay, at least for now. "I won't forget how my mom cried hysterically when she heard my voice. I could only tell her not to worry, that I'm treating the wounded, that I'm okay, and all of this I did while treating, without stopping."

Dr. A, on the other hand, continues to treat an incomprehensible number of casualties in Kibbutz Be'eri in the afternoon hours, but can barely recover. He treats dozens of wounded and evacuates the dead until the next morning, but remembers almost nothing. These are hours when darkness is already descending, along with immense fatigue. "I'm just empty at this point," he tells me, "I'm treating dozens of casualties and evacuating the dead, but I barely remember anything from the night, I only have a vague memory, for example, of an elderly woman with stab wounds who didn't want to be treated, convoys of civilians with their children. A wounded person with a crushed limb, the dead everywhere. But I'm not really there anymore, I'm with the knowledge that one of my best friends from the unit was killed. I become a ghost."

Chapter 11: Only then I cry

The event of mass casualties, by its nature, includes traumatic stress victim. These are patients who witnessed death, mostly brutal deaths, who themselves were in life-threatening situations, who saw horrors, smelled the burning smell that doesn't leave you for days and weeks afterward. Emergency medical personnel and surgeons treating the wounded themselves cannot attend to the psychological casualties, but these are no less severe injuries, ones that will drag trauma for many years, an insurmountable trauma.

Dr. Hadar Sadeh is a child and adolescent psychiatrist specializing and working in Soroka. Among other things, she is one of the founders of a large center for intervention in mental crisis for children and adolescents in Soroka, as part of a national project. All her training she did in Soroka, from the internship to the end of the residency.

"On Saturday morning, with the news of the terror attack, a mass casualty event was declared, as more and more mental health team members from Soroka were arriving," she writes to me. "The truth is that there was no preparation in advance for the event, not sure it would have prepared us for what we encountered. We thought we were coming to treat the usual cases of anxiety from rocket alerts."

The world of mental health is complex. When you're a surgeon, it's simpler: you see a bullet hole, and you discover its path in the surgery itself. You do a full-body CT scan and discover the injuries and their nature, but who can reconstruct the precise path of the injury to the soul? How do you reach an injured soul and know how to say the right words? And sometimes it's more complex cases, like a patient who arrives in an acute panic response and was at a party, for example, and took drugs. Is his response also related to the effects of the substances he took, or not?

"You can divide the patients who arrived roughly into three main groups," Dr. Sadeh tells me. "At first, survivors from the party came in bad shape, then soldiers appeared, and in the evening hours, civilians from the communities appeared, after being released from the siege there. Many of the patients had combined injuries, various body injuries, and acute stress response," she explains.

How do you treat acute stress response? An acute stress response is one in which the patient presents symptoms of arousal and re-experiences of the event. They constantly talk about the event, repeat things, again and again, persistently. There are also dissociative symptoms. The patient disconnects from emotions, feelings, cognitive frameworks. There are situations where the patient doesn't remember who they are, doesn't speak, and doesn't know how to give information to the medical team.

Treatment needs to be focused. In a mass casualty event, the treatment of anxiety victims is centralized at a specific site. It is usually located in the triage area, but slightly further away, allowing physical access to the injured. The goal is to initiate focused intervention in the treatment itself, to calm, contain, indicate that the event is over, and that the patient is in a safe place. Additionally, it is important to renew the sense of security, address feelings, and restore functionality.

A common technique used, also among medical caregivers in the military, is called "Grounding technique." The therapist asks the patient the most basic questions about themselves, like- where are you? What is your name? What is today's date? Where do you live? and tries to focus them on simple things. The Grounding technique can also be performed at a sensory level, in which case the patient is asked to focus their gaze on a specific point in the room, hold something cool like a drink can, and concentrate on the sensory experience itself.

"I entered such an intervention with a patient," Dr. Sadeh tells me, "he was agitated and restless. He repeatedly tells me an incomprehensible, terrifying story. A story that immediately reminds me of my grandmother's stories who was a Holocaust survivor from Auschwitz. He tells me about his friends, saying they were kidnapped. That they were taken to Gaza. I hear his story and I don't believe it's true. I'm sure it's part of the response to stress, a mechanism familiar to patients. And then he shows me a video of them being kidnapped to Gaza. What am I supposed to say? What therapeutic intervention to do? What I encountered in him at that moment is not written in any book. I never learned about this."

Dr. Sadeh realizes that there's the world they taught her how to treat victims of acute stress reactions, the one written about in books, like how to instill a sense of security in the patient and tell them they are in a safe place, or how to construct the sequence of events - past, present, and future - to create a coherent framework to process. But there's what happens in the field, so different from the books.

"How can I tell someone they're in a safe place when they laugh at me and tell me about some safe place I'm talking about, at the same time terrorists could enter here and shoot us?" she asks. "And how can I build the past, present, and future when there's so much uncertainty? When we don't know where family members are and what their fate is, when it's unclear if we should stay there or return to the kibbutz?"

And above all, she notes the fact that as a therapist, you are supposed to provide hope to the despairing patient. "And it's very difficult for me to provide hope. Because I didn't feel it myself. The experience was that our treatment protocols 'disappeared'. Not relevant. There's something much bigger going on here. We worked with therapeutic intuition, with an emphasis on strengthening the internal forces of our patients."

A survivor from one of the kibbutzim told Dr. Sadeh that during the time their house was on fire and they were trapped in the safe room, she felt terrible about not being able to lift her young daughters towards the window to breathe air. Dr. Sadeh tried to comfort her and was impressed by her ability to mediate the event to her daughters and manage to function amidst the chaos. This, for example, is reframing work, a strategy designed to help the patient look at a certain experience from a different, more positive angle.

"Much of our work in triage that day was focused on basic humanity rather than therapy. For example, taking care of people's clean clothes. Giving blanket to the soldier who was in shock, connecting between family members in different triage stations. Providing a response to the families of the missing who arrived at the triage with pictures of their loved ones, channeling their anger and frustration from the chaos, sometimes towards us. Staying with children who arrived alone, with gunshot wounds, while their parents died next to them, just so they wouldn't be alone." And the stories keep flowing that day, along with the feeling that the first thing to do is to be humane. Before the protocol. Before therapeutic intervention.

And the treatment team sees it all. It starts with emotional detachment, like little children coming from the kibbutzim in the periphery. For example, a girl who lost her mother and arrived alone with a gunshot wound, smiled and said "everything's fine." Such a girl needs daily intervention from a skilled child psychologist to be able to share the sequence of events she experienced. It continues with catatonia, like an anonymous soldier arriving at triage in a severe dissociative state, not moving, not speaking, therefore unidentifiable, and he neither eats nor drinks. "I only notice occasionally that he's crying," Dr. Sadeh says, "despite all attempts at intervention, nothing seems to help, not even medication and muscle injections." Only a day later, the same soldier manages to be more organized and starts talking. The family comes to be by his side, and he is discharged home.

The hardest stories are about shattered hope. About families who in despair believed that the patient lying in the ICU unit is their injured son, who never left his bedside even for a moment, as Dr. Amit Frenkel remembers, who managed the mas casualty event in Soroka and cannot forget these cases. "I'll never forget this family, who came sat by the injured's bed, praying for his recovery. Only after some inquiries and more than a day later, we discovered that the injured lying in the same bed is not the son of the parents sitting next to him, but someone else, and they were informed of their son's death identified elsewhere on the premises."

The hours are long, the evening descends, and Dr. Sadeh draws a little comfort from her friends and colleagues in the team, who remain with her to perform interventions and treat couples. She struggles to contain the horrors, and despair fills her completely if she couldn't lean on the friends with her, even in the small hours of the night. "We're also trying to contain the team in triage, which went through a week of indescribable mental difficulty. I receive requests from the teams, like a nurse who comes to me in tears and asks for medication because she doesn't think she'll be able to sleep at home after what she saw and heard in triage."

At a certain point in the early morning, couples arrive at triage who were held by Hamas for long hours. They tell Dr. Sadeh an amazing story, of determination, courage, resilience, and bravery. They tell how they managed to convince Hamas militants not to harm them, and the story itself paints a slightly brighter hue on the day, suddenly giving meaning to the possibility that is different from murder, injuries, and kidnappings - the miraculous survival. The therapists even laugh a little with the couples, who are currently concerned about the electricity in the apartment where they were held and about the meat worth thousands of shekels they have in the freezer that may spoil, "but from all the horror stories I heard, I barely managed to gather hope from this touching story of the surviving couple," she confesses.

Only after long hours, Dr. Sadeh enters her car, on her way home to her children. She managed to maintain professionalism for so long, on emotional appeals, on absorbing the stories and the wounded and the cases that really cannot be contained without something breaking in. Because ultimately, it's impossible that it won't penetrate, like a splinter from a grenade explosion, which remains and wounds you. And only then, when she's alone in the car, she bursts into tears that last the whole way home.

Chapter 12: Pink nail polish

As the evening descends, Sheba Medical Center still buzzes with activity. Despite receiving fewer casualties compared to hospitals in the south, it remains a tertiary trauma center, handling dozens of severe injuries. Operating rooms are packed, the triage lobby is filled with staff, and the emergency department is bustling.

Rotem juggles between the new intense care cases and the old ones. "I try to constantly connect all this chaos with my family. It's been hours since we heard anything from Shira, my cousin, in Nahal Oz. But then another wounded person arrives, caught in gunfire and RPG attacks, so we don't rest for a moment."

She rushes between patients, tending to bleeding wounds, and continues triage work even in the intense care area. The chaos doesn't relent. Helicopters land, surgeries continue, and the hospital operates at full capacity. Meanwhile, during these hours, Dr. Yoram Klein, with the help of Batya Segal, manages the emergency room, admitting many wounded from the south to the operating rooms, the ICU, and the triage.

"Around 5 p.m., I receive a call from a family member," Rotem recounts. "She tells me that Nahal Oz base is completely ablaze, the armory is burning, it's not clear if there are any survivors. And I'm torn. I see all the wounded filling the triage, and I understand that we still need active hands, but on the other hand, I can't take it anymore. The sky is falling on me. I know I have to go to my family, to my sister, to help her, to see what's happening with my cousin, my sister's daughter."

The head nurse of the intensive care unit sees Rotem and understands her without words. She releases her to go home. Rotem leaves details of Shira in the missing persons system, in case she's found, and speeds to her sister's house.

Rotem finds her sister at home, beside herself with worry. It's been hours since they had any contact with Shira, and rumors of the massacre in the south and the complete burning of Nahal Oz base leave them in deep anxiety. Breathless. Shira's father isn't home; he's on his way to the south with the family car. He decided to go alone, to the base, to search for his daughter.

***

Soroka Hospital, late in the evening. The lobby of the triage is filled with people. This is the stage where the injured continue to arrive, but also the families who have managed to escape the turmoil in the border settlements begin to arrive also.

Dr. Ella Shaier finds a few minutes to step out of the emergency rooms that have been working without pause until that hour. "I worked on autopilot in the emergency room, not really aware of the situation outside," she remembers. On that day, over 120 severely injured patients were treated in Soroka's special trauma room, in addition to the hundreds of other casualties who were referred for triage, and she was constantly busy stabilizing their condition. "But when I stepped out to the triage area, outside, I felt that until then I wasn't really connected to the world outside. Only then did the signal drop. Suddenly, I see all the people who came from the settlements and kibbutzim. I see people who hid, broken and shattered, numb, people who lost their homes, lost friends, lost their children. The entrance to the triage resonated with me, the people I saw were in so many forms of chaos. And precisely this event—the exit from the emergency room, and seeing the world outside, or more accurately, the world that was destroyed outside—that's the event that broke me personally."

Meanwhile, Iris, the nurse, and Dr. Yael continue to move together between triage, operating rooms, and the expansion area outside. Throughout the day, there was a tremendous effort to try and identify all the unidentified patients who arrived. "We brought medical students who went to all the departments, trying to search for signs on patients, like tattoos, other identifying marks, and so on. We also went through the operating rooms and the emergency rooms and took pictures of the faces of unidentified patients because families were searching for their loved ones," she recounts. Outside the hospital, hundreds of volunteers arrive, distributing tables with food and drinks, and Iris's heart warms from the collective effort of everyone. "And then I receive a call to quickly come to the pediatric triage, there is a difficult event, and the staff needs help."

On that same day, the pediatric triage at Soroka witnessed difficult scenes, but the nine-month-old twins who arrived for triage after being rescued from the kibbutz where their parents were murdered were one of the toughest sights, leaving the staff in absolute shock. "I arrive at the pediatric triage, and there are two small babies, boys, with blue eyes. Barely a year old. We know nothing about them, except what the rescue team tells us: that their parents were murdered, and they were found alone in the house, abandoned, without food or drink for 11 hours. And I don't know if they need a pacifier or not, what their names are, what they eat, and they cry all the time."

Iris and the medical team try to locate family members. The babies are from Kibbutz Kfar Aza. During the verification process, they realize they have an aunt and uncle living in the center of the country, and grandparents who still don't know anything. Until the initial contact is made, two medical students volunteer to hold the twins in their arms, to comfort and hug them, to check that everything is medically okay. At one in the morning, the aunt arrives, crying. "We, the staff, understand what these twins finally have a name, and that's one of the things that never leaves me. That leaves me speechless," Iris says. She continued with the big triage, only after she saw that the family of the little twins, who were left orphans, arrived to take care of them, and after she completed a support conversation with the nursing and medical staff.

At about this point, Dr. Frenkel, who until now was responsible for managing this huge mass casualty event, transitions from managing the emergency service to a role where he deals with day-to-day, a physician in the ICU unit. "I shower and go to treat severely injured patients hospitalized in Soroka's intensive care unit. I know I will stay there all night, and it's time to make another decision we make that day: to expand the intensive care unit with six additional beds already available in the standby bay for emergency situations. And on the way there, to intensive care, I am exposed to heartbreaking scenes, families who come in droves to the hospital and try to find family members who haven't responded since the morning. People are wandering everywhere with leaflets, names, signs, trying to locate the child, the girl, the husband, the wife, the grandparents."

***

The night descends on Israel. The news editions that worked since six-thirty in the morning continue to report incessantly on the dimensions of the disaster. On the news ticker constantly appears updates about dozens of fatalities, and for those who remained at home on that day and were not at the hospital or in the places where the massacre took place, there is a feeling that the numbers are much larger, just not clear by how much. Only then do stories about the extent of destruction and devastation, about dozens of houses going up in flames, and about charred bodies scattered in the area in indiscernible dimensions, start to emerge. And then the data about the kidnappings also emerges.

And what initially seemed like a small number of kidnapping is becoming increasingly incomprehensible as the hours pass. It will take days until the total number is understood—over two hundred abducted—but videos of horrifying kidnapping, not one or two, but dozens, are already circulating on various networks. And there is a feeling that someone has taken our heart and crushed it with a sledgehammer, that it's hard for us to breathe.

Shira's father arrives at Nahal Oz base. It's eight in the evening, he wanders with the flashlight of his cell phone and searches for his daughter- a beautiful soldier with a pink nail polish and blue eyes like the ocean. On the way to the base, he sees the gates of hell: burning cars, bodies lying on the side of the road, everything charred and rising smoke, and the base itself—the pastoral place he knows from the Saturdays when he visited Shira—filled with the heavy smell of smoke. There are groups of soldiers scanning the area, and dozens of bodies are scattered—bodies of soldiers and soldiers shot at close range. It's already very dark, and he goes room by room, with the flashlight of the iPhone, shouting his daughter's name, Shira, Shira, answer. It's Dad. The ammunition depot located next to the base is completely on fire, barely possible to approach it. In the kitchenette, the bodies of wounded soldiers are lying, and he looks for the girls' quarters, scans every possible place. And then he sees the body of a female soldier. And she has hair like Shira's, and a pink nail polish, and he shouts to the soldiers to come and help him carry his daughter's body, and he calls his wife and family, and informs them, I found her. I found Shira.

The last chapter:
Holocaust

It's 3 a.m. Even if the skies were adorned with stars on that same night, they would have been starless. And even though less than a day has passed since six thirty in the morning, when everything began, in reality, an entire lifetime has passed, spanning many generations. And even if millions of words were written and will be written, and thousands of books and investigations will be conducted — nothing can describe what happened on the morning of October 7th.

Camp Shoora is a military base located in the center of the country, responsible, among other things, for caring for the fallen of the State of Israel. Rotem is now leaving her sister's house for the base. Upon entering the base, she sees a lieutenant colonel, and tells him that she is waiting for her brother-in-law, which is supposed to arrive with the body of her niece, Shira, from the Nahal Oz base.

"These are probably the first bodies from the front," the officer says to her, and she does not understand what he means, how many bodies are we talking about? He points without saying at all the trucks and containers around. "It's all full of bodies," he says. Rotem looks around. An incomprehensible amount of containers loaded with bodies. Hundreds of bodies. And the containers never end. "I collapse on the floor, suddenly realizing that my personal Holocaust is intertwined with the Holocaust that befell the on our entire nation."

She finishes her cigarette, with me on the balcony, and we both fall silent. "You know," she adds, "it didn't end that day. Only after two days did we find out that it wasn't Shira's body at all. Shira was finally identified elsewhere on the base, from the remnants of the D.N.A. It's impossible to describe what we went through. These were days that passed like a mountain railway to hell," she concludes.

Our eyes are already dry from tears, only darkness outside, like in our hearts. Like the darkness in the heart of the family of Amit, the paramedic from Be'eri, whose body was only recovered two days later, with a bullet in her leg, a tourniquet Amit placed in her final moments, a bullet in her head, and rescue vests stained with blood.

And the silence of both of us — Rotem and me — reminds me of Yael's last conversation with her husband, Dr. Eitan Ne'eman, who enlisted in combat on October 7th and was killed two days later. "When I asked him in those hours what was happening, and when he answered me that he was on his way to the commando unit where he volunteered as a doctor, I knew deep down that he would not return, and when I talked to him and said to him, Eitan, take care of yourself, he did not answer me, just smiled and remained silent. I felt the smile through the line, and I knew."

His team members told Yael that the day before he was killed in an encounter with terrorists, on Monday evening, he looked at the sky at night and told them that he was not afraid to die. Someone immortalized him in the last picture of his life, putting on tefillin in the street, as the morning twilight illuminated him. Like all the truly beautiful things, which were revealed in their inconsiderate time, and left an immense void that cannot be filled, like the voice of Amit, the paramedic from Be'eri. When I searched for old videos of hers, I came across a video, from about a year and a half ago, in which she sang on the eve of Memorial Day. These were the words of the song "Longing" by Idan Raichel, and her voice was deep, warm, and greater than life:

"With everything closed to me,
 I soar on the wind
On the wings of all the years.
Secrets and lies.
The wounded heart,
Waiting by the warmth.
Longing."

And I heard, and I learned, and I longed to know Amit, Eitan, Daniel - who was also murdered, the rescue personnel who sacrificed their souls, some in the burning ambulance and some in combat, some in kibbutzim and some in the front lines - who healed until their last moment, and sacrificed their lives, and their families measure the weight of the leaking heart, the heaviness of longing, and nothing will ever be as it was.

And Amit will no longer be the radiant-faced doctor she dreamed to be, and Eitan will no longer save children and babies from the abyss of death, and Shira, the soldier from Nahal Oz, will not be a nurse like Rotem. And only if Amit's father, to whom she had been connected all her life, could feel his daughter resting beside him, in the cemetery, side by side.

And there is no more light in the world, only the glow of those who lit up in the darkness.

List of participants

Dr. A' - Physician in an elite unit in the IDF

Noam Esh Zuntz - Medical student

Menachem Blumenthal - Paramedic, Magen David Adom (MDA)

Noam Barel - Military paramedic, Kerem Shalom Base

Dr. Efrat Bron Harlev – Pediatrician and pediatric intensive care physician, head of Schneider Children's Medical Center

Dr. Ron Berant – Pediatrician and the head of pediatric emergency medicine department, Schneider Children's Medical Center

Noemie Dray - Medic, United Hatzalah

Hani Vaknin - Medic, United Hatzalah

Rotem Zelman - Intensive care and trauma nurse, Sheba Medical Center

Aliza Lev - Social worker, Barzilai Medical Center

Haviva Mann - Sister of Amit Mann (deceased), who was a paramedic in Kibbutz Be'eri

Avi Markus - Paramedic, United Hatzalah

Yael Ne'eman - Widow of Dr. Eitan Naaman (deceased), who was a pediatric intensive care specialist at Soroka Hospital

Batya Segal - Trauma coordinator nurse, Sheba Medical Center

Dr. Michael Segal - Pediatric surgeon, Schneider Children's Medical Center

Dr. Rafi Strugo - Internal medicine and emergency medicine specialist, chief physician, MDA

Dr. Zaki Assi - Senior pediatric surgeon and general surgeon, Head of pediatric surgery department, Soroka Hospital

Dr. Amit Frenkel - Anesthesia and intensive care specialist, head of the Unit for Identifying and Managing Patients at Risk, and head of the MCI, Soroka Hospital

Dr. Yoram Klein - General surgery and trauma specialist, head of the Trauma and Critical Surgery Unit at Sheba Medical Center

Iris Raz - Nurse, midwife, and psychotherapist, Resilience Unit ("Hosen"), Soroka Hospital

Dr. Ela Shaier - Internal medicine and emergency medicine specialist, Soroka Hospital

Dr. Hadar Sadeh - Child and Adolescent psychiatrist, Soroka Hospital

Prof. Eyal Sheiner - Gynecology and obstetrics specialist, director of Women's and Maternity Department B, Soroka Hospital

Made in the USA
Las Vegas, NV
16 May 2024

90011590R00074